Seidel's

PHYSICAL EXAMINATION
Handbook

EIGHTH EDITION

Jane W. Ball, RN, DrPH, CPN
Trauma Systems Consultant
American College of Surgeons
Gaithersburg, Maryland

Joyce E. Dains, DrPH, JD, RN, FNP-BC
Advanced Practice Nursing
  Program Director
The University of Texas
M. D. Anderson Cancer Center
Houston, Texas

John A. Flynn, MD, MBA, MEd
Clinical Director and Professor
  of Medicine
Division of General Internal
  Medicine
The Johns Hopkins University
School of Medicine
Baltimore, Maryland

Barry S. Solomon, MD, MPH
Assistant Professor of Pediatrics
Medical Director, Harriet Lane
  Clinic
Division of General Pediatrics
  and Adolescent Medicine
The Johns Hopkins University
School of Medicine
Baltimore, Maryland

Rosalyn W. Stewart, MD, MS, MBA
Assistant Professor of Pediatrics
  and Medicine
Department of Internal Medicine
  and Pediatrics
The Johns Hopkins University
School of Medicine
Baltimore, Maryland

Reviewer
Susan D. Rymer, MSN, RN
Assistant Professor
School of Nursing
Bellin College
Green Bay, Wisconsin

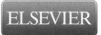

ELSEVIER
MOSBY

3251 Riverport Lane
St. Louis, Missouri 63043

SEIDEL'S PHYSICAL EXAMINATION HANDBOOK   ISBN: 978-0-323-16953-0

Notices

Knowledge and best practice in this field are constantly changing. As new research and experience broaden our understanding, changes in research methods, professional practices, or medical treatment may become necessary.

Practitioners and researchers must always rely on their own experience and knowledge in evaluating and using any information, methods, compounds, or experiments described herein. In using such information or methods, they should be mindful of their own safety and the safety of others, including parties for whom they have a professional responsibility.

With respect to any drug or pharmaceutical products identified, readers are advised to check the most current information provided (i) on procedures featured or (ii) by the manufacturer of each product to be administered to verify the recommended dose or formula, the method and duration of administration, and contraindications.

It is the responsibility of practitioners, relying on their own experience and knowledge of their patients, to make diagnoses, to determine dosages and the best treatment for each individual patient, and to take all appropriate safety precautions.

To the fullest extent of the law, neither the Publisher nor the authors, contributors, or editors, assume any liability for any injury and/or damage to persons or property as a matter of products liability, negligence or otherwise, or from any use or operation of any methods, products, instructions, or ideas contained in the material herein.

International Standard Book Number: 978-0-323-16953-0

Executive Content Strategist: Kristin Geen
Content Manager: Jamie Randall
Associate Content Development Specialist: Melissa Rawe
Publishing Services Manager: Deborah L. Vogel
Project Manager: Pat Costigan
Designer: Paula Catalano

Printed in the United States of America

Last digit is the print number: 9 8 7 6 5 4 3 2

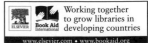

Preface

Seidel's Physical Examination Handbook, eighth edition, is a portable clinical reference on physical examination that is suitable for students of nursing, medicine, chiropractic, osteopathic, and other allied health disciplines, as well as for practicing health care providers. It offers brief descriptions of examination techniques and guidelines on how the examination should proceed, step by step. This handbook is intended to be an aid to review and recall the procedures of physical examination. Because of its brevity specific techniques of history taking by organ system are not described.

The handbook begins with an outline of what information should be obtained for the patient's medical history and review of systems. Subsequent chapters for each of the body systems list equipment needed to perform the examination and present the techniques to be used. Expected and Unexpected Findings follow the description of each technique, presented in distinctive color type for easy recognition. Numerous illustrations interspersed throughout the text reinforce techniques and possible findings. Pediatric examination variations are highlighted in each body systems chapter.

Each chapter offers Aids to Differential Diagnosis and also provides Sample Documentation, which is focused on a specific patient concern to illustrate good documentation practice. Subjective Data and Objective Data are clearly differentiated for each abnormality in the Aids to Differential Diagnosis section of each chapter in the eighth edition.

As in previous editions, separate chapters give an overview of the entire examination for all adults; for infants, children, and adolescents; for older adults; and for healthy females. The final chapter gives guidelines for Reporting and Recording findings.

New chapters in this edition detail the assessment of Vital Signs and Pain, an overview of the older adult examination, and an evaluation for sports participation.

Jane W. Ball
Joyce E. Dains
John A. Flynn
Barry S. Solomon
Rosalyn W. Stewart

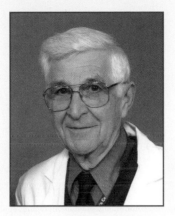

We dedicate the eighth edition of this text to our colleague, Henry M. Seidel, MD, who passed away in 2010. For seven editions, the text has been known as *Mosby's Physical Examination Handbook*. In Henry's honor and memory, we have renamed it *Seidel's Physical Examination Handbook*. Henry spent all of his professional life (except for time served in the U.S. Army), from college through his appointment as Professor Emeritus of Pediatrics, at The Johns Hopkins University. He received numerous awards and a named scholarship at The Johns Hopkins University, testimony of his service at the bedside, in the lecture and seminar rooms, and as Associate Dean for Student Affairs in the School of Medicine. As an original author, we are indebted to him as he contributed greatly to the initial text design as well as to its ongoing development. He understood the importance of communication, sensitivity, and connection with patients, and he was able to share these concepts during the initial book development. He often reminded us that human interaction, sensitivity during history taking, and excellent physical examination skills enable health professionals to understand a patient and develop a healing relationship.

This text was one of the earliest collaborations of a physician and nurse author team, in this case to develop a text targeted to students of medicine, nursing, and other allied health professions. Henry's vision for this text meshed with those of the nurse authors, as well as that of William Benedict, MD, the fourth original author. Through Henry's leadership and collaboration, the authors were able to shape this text and share these important values with students. Henry also wisely planned to have the text's vision remain on course by identifying Barry, John, and Rosalyn, the current physician authors, to continue that vision. We hope we have fulfilled his vision with this edition.

Contents

CONTENTS

CHAPTER 1

The History

BUILDING THE HISTORY

The following outline of a patient history is a guideline and should not be considered a rigid structure. You are beginning your relationship with the patient at this point. Take care with this relationship. Choose a comfortable setting and help the patient get settled. Maintain eye contact and use a conversational tone. Begin by introducing yourself and explaining your role. Help the patient understand why you are building the history and how it will be used. Use open-ended questions to begin and explore responses with additional questions: where, when, what, how, and why. Be sensitive to the patient's emotions. Avoid confrontation and leading questions.

CHIEF CONCERN

- Problem or symptom: reason for visit
- Duration of problem
- Other concerns: secondary issues, fears, concerns, what made patient seek care
- Always consider why this particular problem may be affecting this particular patient at this time. Why did this patient succumb to a risk or an exposure when others similarly exposed did not?

HISTORY OF PRESENT ILLNESS

When more than one problem is identified, address each problem separately.

- Chronologic ordering: sequence of events patient has experienced
- State of health just before onset of present problem
- Complete description of first symptom: time and date of onset, location, movement
- Possible exposure to infection or toxic agents
- If symptoms are intermittent, describe typical attack: onset, duration, symptoms, variations, inciting factors, exacerbating factors, relieving factors
- Impact of illness: on lifestyle, on ability to function; limitations imposed by illness
- "Stability" of problem: intensity, variations, improvement, worsening, staying the same
- Immediate reason for seeking attention, particularly for long-standing problem

- Review of appropriate system when there is a disturbance of a particular organ or system
- Medications: current and recent, dosage of prescriptions, nonprescription medications
- Use of complementary or alternative therapies and medications; home remedies
- At conclusion, review of chronology of events for each problem: patient's confirmations and corrections

MEDICAL HISTORY

- Hospitalizations and/or surgery (including outpatient surgery): dates, hospital, diagnosis, complications, injuries, disabilities
- Major childhood illnesses: measles, mumps, pertussis, varicella, scarlet fever, rheumatic fever
- Major adult illnesses: tuberculosis, hepatitis, diabetes mellitus, hypertension, myocardial infarction, tropical or parasitic diseases, other infections
- Serious injuries: traumatic brain injury, liver laceration, spinal injury, fractures
- Immunizations: polio, diphtheria, pertussis, tetanus toxoid, hepatitis B, measles, mumps, rubella, *Haemophilus influenzae*, varicella, influenza, hepatitis A, meningococcal, human papillomavirus, pneumococcal, zoster, cholera, typhus, typhoid, anthrax, smallpox, bacille Calmette-Guérin, last purified protein derivative (PPD) or other skin tests, unusual reaction to immunizations
- Medications: past, current, and recent medications (dosage, nonprescription medications, vitamins); complementary and herbal therapies
- Allergies: drugs, foods, environmental allergens along with the allergic reaction (e.g., rash, anaphylaxis)
- Transfusions: reason, date, and number of units transfused; reaction, if any
- Mental health: mood disorders, psychiatric therapy or medications
- Recent laboratory tests: glucose, cholesterol, Pap smear/human papillomavirus (HPV), HIV, mammogram, colonoscopy or fecal occult blood test, prostate-specific antigen

FAMILY HISTORY

The genetic basis for a patient's response to risk or exposure may determine whether the patient becomes ill when others do not.
- Relatives with similar illness
- Immediate family: ethnicity, health, cause of and age at death
- History of disease: heart disease, high blood pressure, hypercholesterolemia, cancer, tuberculosis, stroke, epilepsy, diabetes, gout, kidney disease, thyroid disease, asthma and other allergic states, forms of arthritis, blood diseases, sexually transmitted diseases, other familial diseases

- Spouse and children: age, health
- Hereditary disease: history of grandparents, aunts, uncles, siblings, cousins; consanguinity

PERSONAL AND SOCIAL HISTORY

- Cultural background and practices, birthplace, where raised, home environment as youth, education, position in family, marital status or same-sex partner, general life satisfaction, hobbies, interests, sources of stress, religious preference (religious or cultural proscriptions concerning medical care)
- Home environment: number of individuals in household, pets, economic situation
- Occupation: usual work and present work if different, list of job changes, work conditions and hours, physical or mental strain, duration of employment; present and past exposure to heat and cold, industrial toxins; protective devices required or used; military service
- Environment: home, school, work, structural barriers if physically disabled, community services utilized; travel and other exposure to contagious diseases, residence in tropics; water and milk supply, other sources of infection when applicable
- Current health habits and/or risk factors: exercise; smoking (pack years: packs per day × duration); salt intake; obesity/weight control; diet; alcohol intake: (amount/ day), duration; CAGE or TACE question responses (see Appendix on special histories); illicit drugs and methods (e.g., injection, ingestion, sniffing, smoking, or use of shared needles)
- Exposure to chemicals, toxins, poisons, asbestos, or radioactive material at home or work and duration; caffeine use (cups/glasses/day)
- Sexual activity: contraceptive or barrier protection method used; past sexually transmitted infection; treatment
- Screen for domestic or partner violence: see Appendix on special histories
- Complementary and alternative health and medical systems: history and current use
- Religious preference: religious proscriptions concerning medical care
- Concerns about cost of care, health care coverage

REVIEW OF SYSTEMS

It is unlikely that all questions in each system will be asked on every occasion. The following questions are among those that should be asked, particularly at the first interview:

- General constitutional symptoms: fever, chills, malaise, easily fatigued, night sweats, weight (average, preferred, present, change over a specified period and whether this change was intentional)
- Skin, hair, and nails: rash or eruption, itching, pigmentation or texture change; excessive sweating, unusual nail or hair growth

- Head and neck: frequent or unusual headaches, their location, dizziness, syncope; brain injuries, concussions, loss of consciousness (momentary or prolonged)
- Eyes: visual acuity, blurring, double vision, light sensitivity, pain, change in appearance or vision; use of glasses/contacts, eye drops, other medication; history of trauma, glaucoma, familial eye disease
- Ears: hearing loss, pain, discharge, tinnitus, vertigo
- Nose: sense of smell, frequency of colds, obstruction, nosebleeds, postnasal discharge, sinus pain
- Throat and mouth: hoarseness or change in voice; frequent sore throats, bleeding or swelling of gums; recent tooth abscesses or extraction; soreness of tongue or buccal mucosa, ulcers; disturbance of taste
- Lymphatic: enlargement, tenderness, suppuration
- Chest and lungs: pain related to respiration, dyspnea, cyanosis, wheezing, cough, sputum (character and quantity), hemoptysis, night sweats, exposure to tuberculosis; last chest radiograph
- Breasts: development, pain, tenderness, discharge, lumps, galactorrhea, mammograms (screening or diagnostic), breast biopsies
- Heart and blood vessels: chest pain or distress, precipitating causes, timing and duration, relieving factors, palpitations, dyspnea, orthopnea (number of pillows), edema, hypertension, previous myocardial infarction, exercise tolerance (flights of steps, distance walking), past electrocardiogram and cardiac tests
- Peripheral vasculature: claudication (frequency, severity), tendency to bruise or bleed, thromboses, thrombophlebitis
- Hematologic: anemia, any known blood cell disorder
- Gastrointestinal: appetite, digestion, intolerance of any foods, dysphagia, heartburn, nausea, vomiting, hematemesis, bowel regularity, constipation, diarrhea, change in stool color or contents (clay, tarry, fresh blood, mucus, undigested food), flatulence, hemorrhoids, hepatitis, jaundice, dark urine; history of ulcer, gallstones, polyps, tumor; previous radiographic studies, sigmoidoscopy, colonoscopy (where, when, findings)
- Diet: appetite, likes and dislikes, restrictions (because of religion, allergy, or other disease), vitamins and other supplement, caffeine-containing beverages (coffee, tea, cola); food diary or daily listing of food and liquid intake as needed
- Endocrine: thyroid enlargement or tenderness, heat or cold intolerance, unexplained weight change, polydipsia, polyuria, changes in facial or body hair, increased hat and glove size, skin striae
  - Male patients: puberty onset, erections, emissions, testicular pain, libido, infertility
  - Female patients: menses onset, regularity, duration, amount of flow; dysmenorrhea; last period; intermenstrual discharge or bleeding; itching; date of last Pap smear/HPV test; age at menopause; libido; frequency of intercourse; sexual difficulties

- Pregnancy: infertility; gravidity and parity (G = number of pregnancies, P = number of childbirths, A = number of abortions/ miscarriages, L = number of living children); number and duration of each pregnancy, delivery method; complications during any pregnancy or postpartum period; use of oral or other contraceptives
- Genitourinary: dysuria, flank or suprapubic pain, urgency, frequency, nocturia, hematuria, polyuria, hesitancy, dribbling, loss in force of stream, passage of stone; edema of face, stress incontinence, hernias, sexually transmitted infection
- Musculoskeletal: joint stiffness, pain, restriction of motion, swelling, redness, heat, bony deformity, number and pattern of joint involvement
- Neurologic: syncope, seizures, weakness or paralysis, problems with sensation or coordination, tremors
- Mental health: depression, mania, mood changes, difficulty concentrating, nervousness, tension, suicidal thoughts, irritability, sleep disturbances

CONCLUDING QUESTIONS

- Is there anything else that you think would be important for me to know?
- If there are several problems: Which concerns you the most?
- If the history is vague, complicated, or contradictory: What do you think is the matter with you, or what worries you the most?

PEDIATRIC VARIATIONS

BUILDING THE HISTORY

These are only guidelines; you are free to modify and add as the needs of your patients and your judgment dictate.

CHIEF CONCERN

A parent or other responsible adult will generally be the major resource. When age permits, however, the child should be involved as much as possible. Remember that every chief concern has the potential of an underlying concern. What really led to your visit? Was it just the sore throat?

RELIABILITY

Note relationship to patient of person who is the resource for history, and record your impression of the competence of that person as a historian.

HISTORY OF PRESENT ILLNESS

Be sure to give a clear chronologic sequence to the story.

THE HISTORY

MEDICAL HISTORY

In general, the age of the patient and the nature of the problem will guide your approach. Clearly, in a continuing relationship, much of what is to be known will already have been recorded. Certainly, different aspects of the history require varying emphasis depending on the nature of the immediate problem. Certain specifics will command attention, including the following:

- Pregnancy/mother's health:
  - Infectious disease; give approximate gestational month
  - Weight gain/edema
  - Hypertension
  - Proteinuria
  - Bleeding; approximate time
  - Eclampsia, threat of eclampsia
  - Special or unusual diet or dietary practices
  - Medications (hormones, vitamins)
  - Quality of fetal movements, time of onset
  - Radiation exposure
  - Prenatal care/consistency
- Birth and perinatal experience:
  - Duration of pregnancy
  - Delivery site
  - Labor: spontaneous/induced, duration, anesthesia, complications
  - Delivery: presentation; forceps/spontaneous; complications
  - Condition at birth: time of onset of cry; Apgar scores, if available
  - Birth weight and, if available, length and head circumference
- Neonatal period:
  - Hospital experience: length of stay, feeding experience, oxygen needs, vigor, color (jaundice, cyanosis), cry. Did infant go home with mother?
  - First month of life: color (jaundice), feeding, vigor, any suggestion of illness or untoward event
- Feeding:
  - Bottle or breast: any changes and why; type of formula, amounts offered/taken, feeding frequency; weight gain
  - Present diet and appetite: introduction of solids, current routine and frequency, age weaned from bottle or breast, daily intake of milk, food preferences, ability to feed self; elaborate on any feeding problems

DEVELOPMENT

Guidelines suggested in Chapter 21 are complementary to the milestones detailed in the following lists. Those included in this section are commonly used, often remembered, and often recorded in "baby books." Photographs also may occasionally be of some help. **NOTE:** It is important to define the growth and developmental status of each child regardless of the particular concern. That status will inform your understanding of the child, and of the particular problem, and will facilitate the institution of a management plan.

- Age when:
  - Held head erect while held in sitting position
  - Sat alone, unsupported
  - Walked alone
  - Talked in sentences
  - Toilet trained
- School: grade, performance, learning and social problems
- Dentition: ages for first teeth, loss of deciduous teeth, first permanent teeth
- Growth: height and weight at different ages, changes in rate of growth or weight gain or loss
- Sexual: present status (e.g., in female patients, time of breast development, nipples, pubic hair, description of menses; in male patients, development of pubic hair, voice change, acne, emissions). Follow Tanner stages of physical sexual maturity development guides.

FAMILY HISTORY

- Maternal gestational history: all pregnancies with status of each, including date, age, cause of death of all deceased siblings, and dates and duration of pregnancy in the case of miscarriages; mother's health during pregnancy
- Age of parents at birth of patient
- Are parents related to each other in any way?

PERSONAL AND SOCIAL HISTORY

- Personal status:
  - School adjustment
  - Nail biting
  - Thumb sucking
  - Breath-holding
  - Temper tantrums
  - Pica
  - Tics
  - Rituals
- Home conditions:
  - Parental occupation(s)
  - Principal caretaker(s) of patient

- Food preparation, routine, family preferences (e.g., vegetarianism), who does preparing
- Adequacy of clothing
- Dependency on relief or social agencies
- Number of persons and rooms in house or apartment
- Sleeping routines and sleep arrangements for child

REVIEW OF SYSTEMS (SOME SUGGESTED ADDITIONAL QUESTIONS OR PARTICULAR CONCERNS)

- Ears: otitis media (frequency, laterality)
- Nose: snoring, mouth breathing
- Teeth: dental care
- Genitourinary: nature of urinary stream, forceful or a dribble
- Skin, hair, nails: eczema or seborrhea

OLDER ADULT VARIATIONS

FUNCTIONAL ASSESSMENT

- Activities of daily living (ADLs): ability to independently perform or amount of assistance needed with the following:
  - Bathing
  - Dressing
  - Toileting
  - Transfers
  - Grooming
  - Feeding
- Instrumental ADLs: ability to independently perform or amount of assistance needed with the following:
  - Administering own medication
  - Grocery shopping
  - Preparing meals
  - Using the telephone
  - Driving and transportation
  - Handling own finances
  - Housekeeping
  - Laundry
- Risk for falls: falls in the past 6 months or year; use of rugs at home
- Cognitive functioning: see Chapter 3

CHAPTER 2

Vital Signs and Pain Assessment

EQUIPMENT

- Thermometer
- Sphygmomanometer
- Stethoscope
- Pain scales

EXAMINATION

Techniques

Findings

VITAL SIGNS

Temperature

Take the temperature with an oral, tympanic, axillary, temporal, or rectal thermometer.

EXPECTED: Temperature range of 97.2° F to 99.9° F (36.2° C to 37.7° C).
UNEXPECTED: Fever, hypothermia.

Pulse Rate

Palpate the radial or brachial pulse to count the heart rate for 30 seconds and multiply by 2. Note the contour and amplitude of the pulsation. See Chapter 12 for rhythm assessment.

EXPECTED: Rate 60 to 90 beats/min, average 70, regular rhythm.
UNEXPECTED: Bradycardia, tachycardia, irregular rhythm.

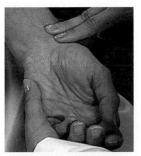
Palpating the radial pulse.

VITAL SIGNS AND PAIN ASSESSMENT

Techniques	Findings
Respiratory Rate Assess the respiratory rate for 30 seconds and multiply by 2. See Chapter 10 to assess the pattern of respirations.	**EXPECTED:** Breathing easy, regular, without distress. Pattern even. Rate 12 to 20 respirations/min. Ratio of respirations to heartbeats about 1:4. **UNEXPECTED:** Tachypnea, bradypnea, dyspnea.
Blood Pressure Measure in both arms at least once annually. Patient's arm should be slightly flexed and positioned or held at the level of the heart.	**EXPECTED:** Less than 120 mm Hg systolic and less than 80 mm Hg diastolic, with pulse pressure of 30 to 40 mm Hg (sometimes to 50 mm Hg). Reading between arms may vary by as much as 10 mm Hg. Prehypertension is now defined as a blood pressure between 120 and 139 mm Hg systolic or 80 and 89 mm Hg diastolic. **UNEXPECTED:** Hypertension (see table below). Unusually low readings should be evaluated for clinical significance.

Classification of Blood Pressure for Adults Ages 18 Years and Older*

Category	Systolic (mm Hg)		Diastolic (mm Hg)
Optimal	Less than 120	and	Less than 80
Prehypertension	120-139	or	80-89
Hypertension[†]			
Stage 1	140-159	or	90-99
Stage 2	160 or higher	or	100 or higher

From National Institutes of Health Publication No. 04-5320, 2004.
*Not taking antihypertensive drugs and not acutely ill. When systolic and diastolic blood pressures fall into different categories, the higher category should be selected to classify the individual's blood pressure status. For example, 160/92 mm Hg should be classified as stage 2 hypertension. In addition to classifying stages of hypertension on the basis of average blood pressure levels, clinicians should specify presence or absence of target organ disease and additional risk factors.
[†]Based on the average of two or more readings taken at each of two or more visits after an initial screening.

Techniques	Findings

Pain Assessment

Explain how to use the pain assessment tool. See figures below. Ask the patient to indicate the pain level at each site and then to describe the pain characteristics. Observe for pain behaviors.

EXPECTED: The patient does not have pain or the painful condition is well managed.

UNEXPECTED: Pain level greater than 3. Pain characteristics such as stabbing, sharp, dull, or aching. Documented pain rating. Behaviors indicating pain such as guarding, facial grimace or other expression of pain, groaning, or rubbing or holding painful site.

VITAL SIGNS AND PAIN ASSESSMENT

PAIN ASSESSMENT TOOLS

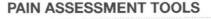

```
0   1   2   3   4   5   6   7   8   9   10
```
No Pain   Moderate   Worst Pain
                         Pain

Numeric Pain Intensity Scale.

No Pain   Worst Pain

Visual analog scale.

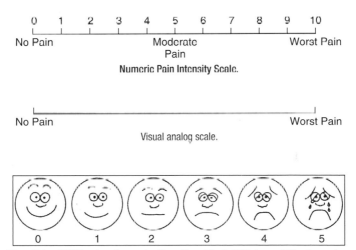

```
   0       1       2       3       4       5
```

Wong-Baker FACES pain rating scale. *From Wong DL et al:* Whaley and Wong's nursing care of infants and children, *ed 7, St Louis, 2003, Mosby.*

VITAL SIGNS AND PAIN ASSESSMENT

PEDIATRIC VARIATIONS

EXAMINATION

Techniques	Findings

Pulse Rate

Palpate the pulse or use a stethoscope to auscultate the apical pulse

EXPECTED:

Age	Beats/min
Newborn	120-170
1 year	80-160
3 years	80-120
6 years	75-115
10 years	70-110

Respiratory Rate

Observe abdominal rise to count the respiratory rate in infants and toddlers.

EXPECTED:

Age	Respirations/min
Newborn	30-80
1 year	20-40
3 years	20-30
6 years	16-22
10 years	16-20
17 years	12-20

UNEXPECTED: Sustained rate higher or lower than expected range.

Measure the Blood Pressure

Select the appropriate size cuff to measure the infant's or child's blood pressure.
- The cuff width should cover approximately 70% of the distance between the shoulder and the elbow.
- The bladder length should be 80% to 100% of the upper arm circumference, and the bladder width should be at least 40% of the arm circumference at the midpoint of the acromion-olecranon distance.

EXPECTED:

For children aged ≥1 year, less than 90th percentile for age, sex, and height (see tables on pp. 13-16).

UNEXPECTED: ≥95th percentile for age, sex, and height.

Blood Pressure Levels for the 90th and 95th Percentiles of Blood Pressure for Boys 1 to 17 Years of Age by Percentile of Height

Age, Years	Blood Pressure Percentile*	Systolic Blood Pressure by Percentile of Height, mm Hg†							Diastolic Blood Pressure by Percentile of Height, mm Hg†						
		5th	10th	25th	50th	75th	90th	95th	5th	10th	25th	50th	75th	90th	95th
1	90th	94	95	97	99	100	102	103	49	50	51	52	53	53	54
	95th	93	99	101	103	104	106	106	54	54	55	56	57	58	58
2	90th	97	99	100	102	104	105	106	54	55	56	57	58	58	59
	95th	101	102	104	106	108	109	110	59	59	59	61	62	63	63
3	90th	100	101	103	105	107	108	109	59	59	60	61	62	63	63
	95th	104	105	107	109	110	112	113	63	63	64	65	66	67	67
4	90th	102	103	105	107	109	110	111	62	63	64	65	66	66	67
	95th	106	107	109	111	112	114	115	66	67	68	69	70	71	71
5	90th	104	105	106	108	110	111	112	65	66	67	68	69	69	70
	95th	103	109	109	112	114	115	116	69	70	71	72	73	74	74
6	90th	105	106	108	110	111	113	113	68	68	69	70	71	72	72
	95th	109	110	112	114	115	117	117	72	72	73	74	75	76	76
7	90th	106	107	109	111	113	114	115	70	70	71	72	73	74	74
	95th	110	111	113	115	117	118	119	74	74	75	76	77	78	78
8	90th	107	109	110	112	114	115	116	71	72	72	73	74	75	76
	95th	111	112	114	116	118	119	120	75	76	77	78	79	79	80
9	90th	109	110	112	114	115	117	118	72	73	74	75	76	76	77
	95th	113	114	116	118	119	121	121	76	76	77	78	79	80	81
10	90th	111	112	114	115	117	119	119	73	73	74	75	76	77	77
	95th	115	116	117	119	121	122	123	77	78	78	79	80	81	82

Continued

Blood Pressure Levels for the 90th and 95th Percentiles of Blood Pressure for Boys 1 to 17 Years of Age by Percentile of Height—Cont'd

Age, Years	Blood Pressure Percentile*	Systolic Blood Pressure by Percentile of Height† mm Hg							Diastolic Blood Pressure by Percentile of Height† mm Hg						
		5th	10th	25th	50th	75th	90th	95th	5th	10th	25th	50th	75th	90th	95th
11	90th	113	114	115	117	119	120	121	74	74	75	76	77	78	78
	95th	117	118	119	121	123	124	125	78	78	79	80	81	82	82
12	90th	115	116	118	120	121	123	123	74	75	75	76	77	78	79
	95th	119	120	122	123	125	127	127	78	79	80	81	82	82	83
13	90th	117	118	120	122	124	125	126	75	75	76	77	78	79	79
	95th	121	122	124	126	128	129	130	79	79	80	82	82	83	83
14	90th	120	121	123	125	126	128	128	75	75	76	78	79	79	80
	95th	124	125	127	128	130	132	132	80	80	81	82	83	84	84
15	90th	122	124	125	127	129	130	131	76	76	77	78	80	80	81
	95th	126	127	129	131	133	134	135	81	81	82	83	84	85	85
16	90th	125	126	128	130	131	133	134	78	78	79	80	81	82	82
	95th	129	130	132	134	135	137	137	82	83	83	84	85	86	87
17	90th	127	128	130	132	134	135	136	80	80	81	82	83	84	84
	95th	131	132	134	136	138	139	140	84	85	86	87	87	88	89

From National High Blood Pressure Education Program Working Group on High Blood Pressure in Children and Adolescents, 2004.

*Blood pressure percentile was determined by a single measurement.

†Height percentile was determined by standard growth curves.

Blood Pressure Levels for the 90th and 95th Percentiles of Blood Pressure for Girls 1 to 17 Years of Age by Percentile of Height

Age, Years	Blood Pressure Percentile*	Systolic Blood Pressure by Percentile of Height† mm Hg							Diastolic Blood Pressure by Percentile of Height† mm Hg						
		5th	10th	25th	50th	75th	90th	95th	5th	10th	25th	50th	75th	90th	95th
1	90th	97	97	98	100	101	102	103	52	53	53	54	55	55	56
	95th	100	101	102	104	105	106	107	56	57	57	58	59	59	60
2	90th	98	99	100	101	103	104	105	57	58	58	59	60	61	61
	95th	102	103	104	105	107	108	109	61	62	62	63	64	65	65
3	90th	100	100	102	103	104	106	106	61	62	62	63	64	64	65
	95th	104	104	105	107	108	109	110	65	66	66	67	68	68	69
4	90th	101	102	103	104	106	107	108	64	64	65	66	67	67	68
	95th	105	106	107	108	110	111	112	68	68	69	70	71	71	72
5	90th	103	103	105	106	107	109	109	66	67	67	68	69	69	70
	95th	107	107	108	110	111	112	113	70	71	71	72	73	73	74
6	90th	104	105	106	108	109	110	111	68	68	69	70	70	71	72
	95th	108	109	110	111	113	114	115	72	72	73	74	74	75	76
7	90th	106	107	108	109	111	112	113	69	70	70	71	72	72	73
	95th	110	111	112	113	115	116	116	73	74	74	75	76	76	77
8	90th	108	109	110	111	113	114	114	71	71	71	72	73	74	74
	95th	112	112	114	115	116	118	118	75	75	75	76	77	78	78
9	90th	110	110	112	113	114	116	116	72	72	72	73	74	75	75
	95th	114	114	115	117	118	119	120	76	76	76	77	78	79	79
10	90th	112	112	114	115	116	118	118	73	73	73	74	75	76	76
	95th	116	116	117	119	120	121	122	77	77	77	78	79	80	80

Continued

Blood Pressure Levels for the 90th and 95th Percentiles of Blood Pressure for Girls 1 to 17 Years of Age by Percentile of Height—Cont'd

Age, Years	Blood Pressure Percentile*	Systolic Blood Pressure by Percentile of Height, mm Hg†							Diastolic Blood Pressure by Percentile of Height, mm Hg†						
		5th	10th	25th	50th	75th	90th	95th	5th	10th	25th	50th	75th	90th	95th
11	90th	114	114	116	117	118	119	120	74	74	74	75	76	77	77
	95th	118	118	119	121	122	123	124	78	78	78	79	80	81	81
12	90th	116	116	117	119	120	121	122	75	75	75	76	77	78	78
	95th	119	120	121	123	124	125	126	79	79	79	80	81	82	82
13	90th	117	118	119	121	122	123	124	76	76	76	77	78	79	79
	95th	121	122	123	124	126	127	128	80	80	80	81	82	83	83
14	90th	119	120	121	122	124	125	125	77	77	77	78	79	80	80
	95th	123	123	125	126	127	129	129	81	81	81	82	83	84	84
15	90th	120	121	122	123	125	126	127	78	78	78	79	80	81	81
	95th	124	125	126	127	129	130	131	82	82	82	83	84	85	85
16	90th	121	122	123	124	126	127	128	78	78	79	80	81	81	82
	95th	125	126	127	128	130	131	132	82	82	83	84	85	86	86
17	90th	122	122	123	125	126	127	128	78	79	79	80	81	81	82
	95th	125	126	127	129	130	131	132	82	83	83	84	85	85	86

From National High Blood Pressure Education Program Working Group on High Blood Pressure in Children and Adolescents, 2004.

*Blood pressure percentile was determined by a single measurement.

†Height percentile was determined by standard growth curves.

Techniques

Findings

Pain Assessment

Observe for pain behaviors using a tool such as the Face, Legs, Activity, Cry, and Consolability (FLACC) Behavioral Pain Assessment Scale when the child is unable to use a self-report pain assessment tool. See FLACC figure below.

UNEXPECTED: The child has pain behaviors such as crying, posturing, restlessness, facial grimace, and is difficult to comfort.

CATEGORIES	SCORING		
	0	1	2
Face	No particular expression or smile	Occasional grimace or frown; withdrawn, disinterested	Frequent to constant frown, clenched jaw, quivering chin
Legs	Normal position or relaxed	Uneasy, restless, tense	Kicking or legs drawn up
Activity	Lying quietly, normal position, moves easily	Squirming, shifting back and forth, tense	Arched, rigid, or jerking
Cry	No cry (awake or asleep)	Moans or whimpers, occasional complaint	Crying steadily, screams or sobs; frequent complaints
Consolability	Content, relaxed	Reassured by occasional touching, hugging, or being talked to; distractable	Difficult to console or comfort

Guidelines for Scoring the FLACC

Face
Score 0 if the patient has a relaxed face, makes eye contact, shows interest in surroundings.
Score 1 if the patient has a worried facial expression, with eyebrows lowered, eyes partially closed, cheeks raised, mouth pursed.
Score 2 if the patient has deep furrows in the forehead, closed eyes, an open mouth, deep lines around nose and lips.

Legs
Score 0 if the muscle tone and motion in the limbs are normal.
Score 1 if the patient has increased tone, rigidity, or tension; if there is intermittent flexion or extension of the limbs.
Score 2 if patient has hypertonicity, the legs are pulled tight, there is exaggerated flexion or extension of the limbs, tremors.

Activity
Score 0 if the patient moves easily and freely, normal activity or restrictions.
Score 1 if the patient shifts positions, appears hesitant to move, demonstrates guarding, a tense torso, pressure on a body part.
Score 2 if the patient is in a fixed position, rocking; demonstrates side-to-side head movement or rubbing of a body part.

Cry
Score 0 if the patient has no cry or moan, awake or asleep.
Score 1 if the patient has occasional moans, cries, whimpers, sighs.
Score 2 if the patient has frequent or continuous moans, cries, grunts.

Consolability
Score 0 if the patient is calm and does not require consoling.
Score 1 if the patient responds to comfort by touching or talking in 30 seconds to 1 minute.
Score 2 if the patient requires constant comforting or is inconsolable.

Interpreting the Behavioral Score
Each category is scored on the 0–2 scale, which results in a total score of 0–10.

0 = Relaxed and comfortable   4–6 = Moderate pain
1–3 = Mild discomfort   7–10 = Severe discomfort or pain or both

Face, Legs, Activity, Cry, and Consolability (FLACC) Behavioral Pain Assessment Scale for nonverbal children. *(From Merkel et al, 1997)*

Techniques	Findings

For nonverbal older children and adults, use the Checklist of Nonverbal Pain Indicators to assess pain behaviors.

Signs	With Movement	At Rest
Vocal Complaints—nonverbal expression of pain demonstrated by moans, groans, grunts, cries, gasps, sighs		
Facial Grimaces and Winces—furrowed brow, narrowed eyes, tightened lips, dropped jaw, clenched teeth, distorted expression		
Bracing—clutching or holding onto siderails, bed, tray table, or affected area during movement		
Restlessness—constant or intermittent shifting of position, rocking, intermittent or constant hand motions, inability to keep still		
Rubbing—massaging affected area		
Vocal Complaints—verbal expression of pain using words, e.g., "ouch" or "that hurts;" cursing during movement, or exclamations of protest, e.g., "stop" or "that's enough."		
TOTAL SCORE		

Instructions: Score a 0 if the behavior was not observed; score a 1 if the behavior was observed even briefly during activity or rest. The total score ranges from 0 to 5.

The Checklist of Nonverbal Pain Indicators with movement and at rest. *(From Feldt, 2000.)*

CHAPTER 3

Mental Status

EQUIPMENT

- Familiar objects (coins, keys, paper clips)
- Paper and pencil

EXAMINATION

Perform the mental status examination throughout the patient interaction. Focus on the patient's alertness, orientation, mood, and cognition or complex mental processes (learning, perceiving, decision making, and memory).

Use a mental status screening examination for health visits when no cognitive, emotional, or behavioral problems are apparent. Information is generally observed during the history in the following areas:

Appearance and behavior

Grooming
Emotional status
Body language

Emotional stability

Mood and feelings
Thought process and content

Cognitive abilities

State of consciousness
Memory
Attention span
Judgment

Speech and language

Voice quality
Articulation
Comprehension
Coherence
Ability to communicate

When concerned about any of the patient's responses or behaviors, ask a family member if the patient has had any problems with the following: remembering important appointments or events, paying bills, shopping independently for food or clothing, taking medication, getting lost while walking or driving, making decisions about daily life, or asking the same thing again and again (Maslow and Mezey, 2008).

MENTAL STATUS

Technique	Findings

Mental Status and Speech Patterns

Observe physical appearance and behavior

- *Grooming*

UNEXPECTED: Poor hygiene; lack of concern with appearance; or inappropriate dress for season, gender, or occasion in previously well-groomed patient.

- *Emotional status*

EXPECTED: Usually friendly and cooperative; expresses concern appropriate for emotional content of topics discussed.

UNEXPECTED: Behavior conveys carelessness, apathy, loss of sympathetic reactions, unusual docility, rage reactions, agitation, or excessive irritability.

- *Body language*

EXPECTED: Erect posture and eye contact (if culturally appropriate).

UNEXPECTED: Slumped posture, lack of facial expression, excessively energetic movements, or constantly watchful eyes.

- *State of consciousness*

EXPECTED: Oriented to person, place, and time; appropriate responses to questions and environmental stimuli.

UNEXPECTED: Disoriented to time, place, or person. Verbal response is confused, incoherent, or inappropriate, or there is no verbal response.

Investigate cognitive abilities

- *Mini-Cog*

Ask patient to remember and immediately repeat three unrelated words (e.g., *red*, *plate*, and *milk*). Ask patient to draw a clock face with numbers, then place hands pointing to the time you specify. Allow 3 minutes. Ask the patient to repeat the three words. Score 1 point for each word recalled.

EXPECTED: All three words are remembered, and the clock face has all numbers in proper position and hands pointing to the specified time.

UNEXPECTED: A score of ≤2 may indicate dementia.

Technique	Findings

Score 2 points when all numbers of the clock face are near the rim, in correct sequence, and hands point to the specified time. Total of 5 points (Doerflinger, 2007).

- *Mini-Mental State Examination (MMSE)*
Use this examination to quantify cognitive function or document changes. See http://www.minimental.com/ to access the full tool.

EXPECTED: Score of 26-30. Score of 21-25 is borderline.
UNEXPECTED: Score ≤20 is associated with dementia.

- *Set test*
Use this test to evaluate mental status as a whole (motivation, alertness, concentration, short-term memory, problem solving). Ask patient to name 10 items in each of 4 groups: fruit, animals, colors, towns, or cities. Give each item 1 point for a maximum of 40 points (Chopard et al, 2007).

EXPECTED: Able to categorize, count, remember items listed. Score of ≥25 points.
UNEXPECTED: Score <15 points. Check for mental changes or cultural, educational, or social factors when score is 15-24.

- *Analogies*
Ask patient to describe analogies: first simple, then more complex
  - What is similar about peaches and lemons, oceans and lakes, trumpet and flute?
  - An engine is to an airplane as an oar is to a _____?
  - What is different about a magazine and a telephone book, or a bush and a tree?

EXPECTED: Correct responses when patient has average intelligence.
UNEXPECTED: Unable to describe similarities or differences.

- *Abstract reasoning*
Ask patient to explain meaning of fable, proverb, or metaphor.
  - A stitch in time saves nine.
  - A bird in the hand is worth two in the bush.
  - A rolling stone gathers no moss.

EXPECTED: Adequate interpretation when patient has average intelligence.
UNEXPECTED: Unable to give adequate explanation.

MENTAL STATUS

Technique	Findings
• *Arithmetic calculations* Ask patient to perform simple calculations without paper and pencil. • 50 – 7, – 7, – 7, etc., until answer is 8. • 50 + 8, + 8, + 8, etc., until answer is 98.	**EXPECTED:** Able to complete with few errors within a minute. **UNEXPECTED:** Unable to perform calculations.
• *Writing ability* Ask patient to write name and address or a phrase you dictate (or if literacy is a problem, draw figures—triangle, circle, square, flower, house, clock face).	**UNEXPECTED:** Omission or addition of letters, syllables, or words; mirror writing; or uncoordinated writing (or figure drawings).
• *Execution of motor skills* Ask patient to do a motor task such as combing hair or putting on lipstick.	**UNEXPECTED:** Inability to complete a task that is not related to paralysis.
• *Memory* *Immediate recall or new learning*: Ask patient to listen to, then repeat, a sentence or series of numbers. *Recent memory*: Ask the patient to remember the four or five objects shown, or give a visually impaired patient four unrelated words with distinct sounds to remember (carpet, iris, bench, fortune). In 10 minutes, ask patient to list objects. *Remote memory*: Ask patient about verifiable past events (e.g., mother's maiden name, name of high school, subject of common knowledge).	**EXPECTED:** *Immediate recall*: Able to repeat sentence or numbers (five to eight numbers forward, four to six numbers backward). *Recent memory*: Able to remember test objects. *Remote memory*: Able to recall verifiable past events. **UNEXPECTED:** Impaired memory. Loss of immediate and recent memory with retention of remote memory.
• *Attention span* Ask patient to follow a series of short commands (e.g., take off all clothes, put on patient gown, sit on examining table), or spell "*world*" forward and backward. Arithmetic calculation is another test of attention span.	**EXPECTED:** Responds to directions appropriately. **UNEXPECTED:** Easy distraction or confusion, negativism.

Technique	Findings
• *Judgment* Explore: • How patient meets social and family obligations, patient's future plans. • Patient's solutions to hypothetical situations (e.g., found stamped envelope or was stopped for running red light).	**EXPECTED:** Able to evaluate situation and provide appropriate response; managing family and business affairs appropriately. **UNEXPECTED:** Response indicating hazardous behavior or inappropriate action.
Observe speech and language • *Voice quality*	**EXPECTED:** Uses inflections, speaks clearly and strongly, is able to increase voice volume and pitch. **UNEXPECTED:** Difficulty or discomfort making laryngeal speech sounds or varying volume, quality, or pitch of speech.
• *Articulation*	**EXPECTED:** Proper pronunciation of consonants; fluent and rhythmic speech; easily expresses thoughts. **UNEXPECTED:** Imperfect or slurring pronunciation, difficulty articulating single speech sound, or speech with hesitancy, stuttering, or repetitions.
• *Comprehension*	**EXPECTED:** Able to follow simple 1- and 2-step instructions.
• *Coherence*	**EXPECTED:** Able to clearly convey intentions or perceptions. **UNEXPECTED:** Circumlocutions, perseveration, flight of ideas or loosening of associations between thoughts, gibberish, neologisms, clang association, echolalia, or unusual sounds may be associated with a psychiatric disorder. Hesitations, omissions, inappropriate word substitutions, circumlocutions, neologisms, disturbance of rhythm or words in sequence may be signs of aphasia.

MENTAL STATUS

MENTAL STATUS

Technique	Findings

Evaluate emotional stability

- *Mood and feelings*

Ask patient how he or she feels, whether feelings are a problem in daily life, and whether he or she has particularly difficult times or experiences.

EXPECTED: Expresses appropriate feelings for the situation.
UNEXPECTED: Unresponsiveness, hopelessness, agitation, aggression, anger, euphoria, irritability, or wide mood swings.

- *Depression screening questions*
  - Over the past 2 weeks, have you felt down, depressed, or hopeless?
  - Over the past 2 weeks, have you felt little interest or pleasure in doing things?

EXPECTED: Negative response to one or both questions.
UNEXPECTED: Positive response to both questions indicates a need to ask more questions about depression symptoms of fatigue, restlessness, and poor concentration.

Ask the patient to choose the best answer for how he or she felt over the previous week.

1. Are you basically satisfied with your life?	YES / NO
2. Have you dropped many of your activities and interests?	YES / NO
3. Do you feel that your life is empty?	YES / NO
4. Do you often get bored?	YES / NO
5. Are you in good spirits most of the time?	YES / NO
6. Are you afraid that something bad is going to happen to you?	YES / NO
7. Do you feel happy most of the time?	YES / NO
8. Do you feel helpless?	YES / NO
9. Do you prefer to stay at home, rather than going out and doing new things?	YES / NO
10. Do you feel you have more problems with memory than most?	YES / NO
11. Do you think it is wonderful to be alive now?	YES / NO
12. Do you feel pretty worthless the way you are now?	YES / NO
13. Do you feel full of energy?	YES / NO
14. Do you feel that your situation is hopeless?	YES / NO
15. Do you think most people are better off than you are?	YES / NO

Correct responses are the following:
 Yes for questions 2, 3, 4, 6, 8, 9, 10, 12, 14, and 15.
 No for questions 1, 5, 7, 11, and 13.
Give one point for each correct answer. A score greater than five suggests depression.

Geriatric Depression Scale. *(From Sheikh and Yesavage, 1986.)*

- *Thought process and content*
  - Ask patient about obsessive thoughts relating to making decisions, fears, or guilt.

EXPECTED: Patient's thought processes can be followed, and ideas expressed are logical and goal directed.

MENTAL STATUS

Technique	Findings
• Ask patient about the need to compulsively repeat actions, check, and recheck (or observe the patient's actions). • Observe sequence, logic, coherence, and relevance of topics. • Does patient have delusions (of grandeur, of being controlled by external force)? Does the patient feel watched, followed, persecuted, or paranoid?	**UNEXPECTED:** Illogical or unrealistic thought processes; blocking or disturbance in stream of thinking. Obsessive thought content, compulsive behavior, phobias, anxieties that interfere with daily life or are disabling. Delusions.

• *Perceptual distortions and hallucinations*
  • Ask patient about any sensations not believed to be caused by external stimuli.
  • Find out when these experiences occur.
	UNEXPECTED: Sensory hallucinations—hears voices, sees vivid images or shadowy figures, smells offensive odors, feels worms crawling on skin.

AIDS TO DIFFERENTIAL DIAGNOSIS

Subjective Data	Objective Data
Dementia	
Forgets significant events; gets lost in familiar areas; unable to manage shopping, food preparation, medications; mood changes (depression, uncharacteristic anger, anxiety, or agitation); apathy.	Impaired memory, social and occupational functioning, and activities of daily living; impaired use of language; progressive deterioration in cognitive function.
Delirium	
Sudden impairment of memory and attentiveness, mood swings, increased or decreased activity.	Altered consciousness; fearful, suspicious; rambling and irrelevant conversation, illogical flow of ideas. Misperceptions, illusions, hallucinations, and delusions; symptoms increase and decrease during the day.

MENTAL STATUS

Subjective Data	Objective Data

Depression

Feels sad, hopeless, worthless; loss of pleasure or interest; insomnia or excessive sleeping; increased or decreased appetite. May have had a loss, change in health status, stressful life event.

Altered mood and affect with extreme sadness, anxiety, irritability; impaired concentration, reduced attention span, indecisiveness, slower thought processes.

Mania

Persistently elevated and expansive mood, hyperactivity, overconfidence, exaggerated view of own abilities.

Increased talkativeness or pressure to keep talking with excessive rhyming, puns, or flight of ideas; impaired attention, judgment, social, occupational, and interpersonal functioning; grandiose or persecutory delusions.

Anxiety disorder

Anxiety or fear that interferes with personal, social, occupational functioning. Panic attacks (palpitations, sweating, shaking, dizziness, nausea, chest pain, abdominal distress); nightmares; flashbacks; poor concentration; sleeps poorly.

Tachycardia, diaphoresis, tremors, impaired attention, ritualized acts performed compulsively.

SAMPLE DOCUMENTATION

Subjective. A 66-year-old woman accompanied by spouse who expresses concern about his wife's memory loss. She got lost in the local shopping mall last week. Previously was a good cook, but over the last few months either does not have necessary ingredients or has difficulty following recipes. Needs help to take correct daily medications. Dresses and undresses self, but needs help to select clothes to wear. Patient recognizes all family members and social contacts, and is able to talk with them.

Objective. Pleasant woman with clear speech, responds to simple questions correctly. Turns to spouse frequently for answers to some history questions. Follows one-step directions, but needs reminder with two-step directions. Immediate and recent memory impaired, but remote memory is intact. Arithmetic calculation impaired. Mini-Cog score = 2, and Set Test score = 14.

PEDIATRIC VARIATIONS

EXAMINATION

Technique	Findings

Mental Status

Use parent's impression of infant's responsiveness to guide your assessment. Questionnaires completed by parents (e.g., Ages and Stages Questionnaire or Parent's Evaluation of Developmental Status) are effective screening tools.

EXPECTED: Infant responds appropriately to parent's voice, is attentive, comforts easily.
Social smile can be elicited; babbling or cooing or language appropriate for age.
Child follows simple directions.
UNEXPECTED: Nonresponsive, inconsolable, combative, lethargic.

MENTAL STATUS

AIDS TO DIFFERENTIAL DIAGNOSIS

Subjective Data	Objective Data

Intellectual Disability

Delayed motor, speech, and language development.

Delayed developmental milestones, impaired cognitive functioning and short-term memory; poor academic performance; lack of motivation.

Autism

Does not make eye contact or point to share experiences with others; resists being held or touched; odd and repetitive behaviors, ritualized play, preoccupation with objects; motor development appropriate for age.

Impaired social interactions and language, odd intonation to speech, pronoun reversal, nonsensical rhyming; lacks awareness of others.

Attention-deficit/hyperactivity

Short attention span, easily distracted, fidgets and squirms, often moving, disruptive behavior, talks excessively, temper outbursts; has problems in more than one setting.

Increased motor activity, difficulty organizing tasks, poor school performance.

CHAPTER 4

Nutrition and Growth and Measurement

EQUIPMENT

- Tape measure with millimeter markings
- Standing platform scale with height attachment
- Scale (kilogram) for weighing infants and children
- Device for measure length of children younger than 2 years
- Stadiometer for measuring height of children
- Calculator
- Skinfold caliper

EXAMINATION

Technique	Findings

Anthropometrics

Measure height and weight

- *Estimate desirable body weight*
Add 10% for large frame; subtract 10% for small frame.

EXPECTED: *Women:* 100 pounds for first 5 feet, plus 5 pounds for each inch thereafter. *Men:* 106 pounds for first 5 feet, plus 6 pounds for each inch thereafter.

- *Calculate percent weight change*

$$\left(\frac{\text{Usual weight} - \text{Current weight}}{\text{Usual weight}} \right) \times 100$$

UNEXPECTED: Weight loss that equals or exceeds 1% to 2% in 1 week, 5% in 1 month, 7.5% in 3 months, 10% in 6 months.

- *Calculate body mass index (BMI)* kg/m^2 *or calculate using pounds by*

$$\left(\frac{\text{Weight in pounds} \times 703}{\text{Height in inches}} \right) \div \begin{array}{l}\text{Height in}\\\text{inches}\end{array}$$

EXPECTED: 18.5-24.9 for men and women.

UNEXPECTED: BMI <18.5 is classified as undernutrition. BMI 25-29.9 is classified as overweight. BMI 30-39.9 is obesity. BMI ≥40 is extreme obesity.

Technique	Findings
Measure waist circumference Indicator of visceral fat. Using a tape measure with millimeter markings, measure waist at high point of iliac crest when patient is standing and at minimal respiration.	**EXPECTED:** Waist circumference <40 inches for men and <35 inches for women. **UNEXPECTED:** Measurements >40 inches in men and >35 inches in women are associated with increased risk for type 2 diabetes, hypertension, and cardiovascular disease.
Calculate waist-to-hip circumference ratio Another measure of fat distribution. Using tape measure with millimeter markings, measure waist at a mid-point between the costal margin and the iliac crest. Then measure hip at the widest part of the gluteal region. Divide waist circumference by hip circumference to obtain the ratio.	**EXPECTED:** Ratio <0.9 in men and <0.8 in women. **UNEXPECTED:** Ratios >1.0 in men and >0.85 in women indicate increased central fat distribution and increased risk for obesity-related disease.

Determine Diet Adequacy

24-hour diet recall

Ask patient to complete 24-hour food and beverage recall. Ask specific questions about method of food preparation, portion sizes, amount of sugar-sweetened beverages, and use of salt or other additives. The U.S. Department of Agriculture ChooseMyPlate.gov website, based on the 2010 *Dietary Guidelines for Americans*, has a useful web-based tool for tracking daily food and beverage intake by food groups (grains, vegetables, fruits, dairy and protein foods; www.supertracker.usda.gov/default.aspx)

EXPECTED: Plate of food should have half fruits and vegetables and half grains and protein. Recommended daily amounts of fruits, vegetables, grains, and protein is based on the individual's age, sex, and level of physical activity. Recommendations can be found at the ChooseMyPlate.gov website.

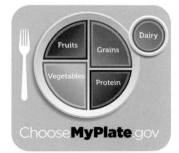

From U.S. Department of Agriculture: ChooseMyPlate, 2013, http://www.choosemyplate.gov.

Technique	Findings

Determine Nutritional Adequacy

Calculate estimates for energy needs

Use actual weight for healthy adults.

Use adjusted weight for obese patients.

Calories	Kcal/kg
Weight loss	25
Weight maintenance	30
Weight gain	35
Hypermetabolic/ malnourished	35-50

Estimate fat intake

Provides 9 calories per gram; present in fatty fish, animal, and some plant products; classified as saturated, trans, monounsaturated, and polyunsaturated.

EXPECTED: 20% to 35% of the daily calories consumed should come from fat.

Estimate protein intake

Provides 4 calories per gram; present in all animal and plant products.

EXPECTED: 10% to 35% of daily calories consumed should come from protein; Recommended Daily Allowance (RDA) goal is 46 g for adult women and 56 g in adult men.

Estimate carbohydrate intake

Provides 4 calories per gram; classified as simple (sugars) or complex (starches and fibers).

EXPECTED: 45% to 65% of the total calories consumed should come from carbohydrates, with selections predominantly coming from complex carbohydrates.

Estimate fiber intake

EXPECTED: Adequate Intake is 25 g/day for adult women and 38 g/day for adult men. Recommended fiber intake ranges from 14 to 31 g/day for children aged 1-18 years.

Technique	Findings

Special Procedures

Measure mid–upper arm circumference (MAC)

Place measuring tape around upper right arm, midway between tips of olecranon and acromial processes. Hold tape snugly and make the reading to nearest 5 mm. This measurement is used along with the triceps skinfold (TSF) thickness to calculate midarm muscle circumference (MAMC).

EXPECTED: Between 10th and 95th percentiles.
UNEXPECTED: <10th or >95th percentile (see table below).

Percentiles for Midarm Circumference (MAC), Midarm Muscle Circumference (MAMC), and Triceps Skinfold (TSF) Thickness

	Men		Women	
Percentile	55-65 yr	65-75 yr	55-65 yr	65-75 yr
MAC, cm				
10th	27.3	26.3	25.7	25.2
50th	31.7	30.7	30.3	29.9
95th	36.9	35.5	38.5	37.3
MAMC, cm				
10th	24.5	23.5	19.6	19.5
50th	27.8	26.8	22.5	22.5
95th	32.0	30.6	28.0	27.9
TSF, mm				
10th	6	6	16	14
50th	11	11	25	24
95th	22	22	38	36

From Frisancho (1981).

Technique	Findings

Measure TSF thickness

Have patient flex right arm at a right angle. Find midpoint between tips of olecranon and acromial processes on the posterior arm, and make a horizontal mark. Then draw a vertical line to intersect. With arm relaxed, use your thumb and forefinger to grasp and lift TSF about ½ inch proximal to intersection marks. Place caliper at skinfold and measure without making an indentation. Make 2 readings to nearest millimeter and derive an average. This measurement is used along with the MAC to calculate MAMC.

EXPECTED: Between 10th and 95th percentiles.
UNEXPECTED: <10th or >95th percentile (see table on p. 31).

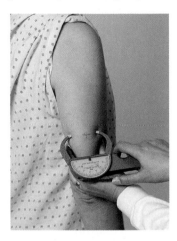

Calculate MAMC

$$MAMC = \{MAC \ (mm) - [3.14 \times TSF \ (mm)]\}$$

Compare measurement with table for percentiles.

EXPECTED: Between 10th and 95th percentiles.

UNEXPECTED: <10th or >95th percentile (see table on p. 31).

Biochemical Measurements

Obtain biochemical measures as indicated

Hemoglobin
Hematocrit
Serum albumin
Transferrin saturation
Serum glucose
Triglycerides
Cholesterol
High-density lipoprotein (HDL) cholesterol
Cholesterol/HDL ratio
Low-density lipoprotein (LDL) cholesterol
Hemoglobin A_1c
Serum folate

EXPECTED: See reference ranges established by your particular laboratory.

AIDS TO DIFFERENTIAL DIAGNOSIS

Subjective Data	Objective Data

Obesity

Excessive caloric intake, weight gain, decrease in physical exercise, recent life change or stress, medications.

BMI—overweight: 25-29.9, obesity: 30-39.9, extreme obesity: ≥40; excess fat located in breasts, buttocks, thighs; may have pale striae or acanthosis nigricans.

Anorexia nervosa

Use of weight-control measures (e.g., voluntary starvation, purging, vomiting, diet pills, laxative abuses, and diuretic use); possible excessive exercise, unusual eating habits.

Failure to maintain weight at 85% of ideal body weight for age and height, BMI ≤17.5; dry skin, lanugo hair, brittle nails, bradycardia, hypothermia, orthostatic hypotension, loss of muscle mass and subcutaneous fat; may have hypoglycemia, elevated liver enzymes, and thyroid hormone abnormalities.

Bulimia

Binge-eating episodes on average of 2 times per week followed by purging (e.g., vomiting, laxatives, diuretics); bloating, fullness, abdominal pain, heartburn.

Body weight may be normal, underweight, or overweight; knuckle calluses, dental enamel erosion, salivary gland enlargement; may have metabolic alkalosis, hypokalemia, or elevated salivary amylase.

Clinical Signs and Symptoms of Various Nutrient Deficiencies

Body Part or System	Sign/Symptom	Deficiency
Eyes	Xerosis of conjunctiva	Vitamin A
	Keratomalacia	Vitamin A
	Bitot spots	Vitamin A
	Corneal vascularization	Riboflavin
Gastrointestinal tract	Nausea, vomiting	Pyridoxine
	Diarrhea	Zinc, niacin
	Stomatitis	Pyridoxine, riboflavin, iron
	Cheilosis	Pyridoxine, iron
	Glossitis	Pyridoxine, zinc, niacin, folate, vitamin B_{12}
		Riboflavin
		Vitamin C
		Protein

Continued

Clinical Signs and Symptoms of Various Nutrient Deficiencies—cont'd

Body Part or System	Sign/Symptom	Deficiency
Skin	Dry and scaling	Vitamin A, essential fatty acids, zinc
	Petechiae/ecchymoses	Vitamin C, vitamin K
	Follicular hyperkeratosis	Vitamin A, essential fatty acids
	Nasolabial seborrhea	Niacin, pyridoxine, riboflavin
	Atopic dermatitis	Niacin, zinc
Hair	Alopecia	Zinc, essential fatty acids
	Easy pluckability	Protein, essential fatty acids
	Lackluster	Protein, zinc
	"Corkscrew" hair	Vitamin C, vitamin A
	Decreased pigmentation	Protein, copper
Extremities	Subcutaneous fat loss	Calories
	Muscle wastage	Calories, protein
	Edema	Protein
	Osteomalacia, bone pain, rickets	Vitamin D
	Arthralgia	Vitamin C
Neurologic	Disorientation	Niacin, thiamin
	Confabulation	Thiamin
	Neuropathy	Thiamin, pyridoxine, chromium
	Paresthesia	Thiamin, pyridoxine, vitamin B_{12}
Cardiovascular	Congestive heart failure, cardiomegaly, tachycardia	Thiamin
	Cardiomyopathy	Selenium

SAMPLE DOCUMENTATION

Subjective. A 45-year-old man with steady weight gain over the past 5 years seeks nutrition counseling for weight-loss plan. Eats three full meals each day with snacking in between; eats breakfast and dinner at home, where wife prepares meals. Often eats lunch (fast foods) on the run. Sugar beverage intake: one or two cans of non-diet soda per day. No regular exercise. Has never kept a meal log. No change in lifestyle; moderate stress.

Objective. Height: 173 cm (68 inches). Weight: 90.9 kg (200 pounds), 123% of desirable body weight; BMI: 30.5; TSF thickness: 20 mm, 90th percentile; MAC: 327.8 mm; MAMC: 26.5 cm, 25th percentile; waist circumference: 42 inches; hip circumference: 41 inches; waist-to-hip ratio: 1.02; 2200 calories daily estimated for appropriate weight loss.

PEDIATRIC VARIATIONS

EXAMINATION

Technique	Findings
Anthropometrics	
Growth assessment	
Measure the length of infants and children until age 2 years. Weigh the child. Calculate BMI starting at 2 years of age. Use growth charts for pediatric patients (available at www.cdc.gov/growthcharts).	**EXPECTED:** Child is following a growth curve pattern for length or height and weight. Length or height and weight are approximately same percentiles. BMI following a growth pattern expected for age.
Measure head circumference	
Wrap tape measure snugly around the head at the occipital protuberance and supraorbital prominence for infants and children younger than 2 years.	**UNEXPECTED:** Head circumference <3rd percentile, or increasing in size at a rate faster than expected for age.
Calculate estimates for energy needs	
• *Pediatric patients*	**EXPECTED:** *Fat intake:* Ages 1-3 years, 30% to 40% of daily calories, ages 4-18 years, 25% to 35% of daily calories. *Protein intake:* Ages 1-3 years, 5% to 20% of daily calories, ages 4-18, 10% to 30%

CHAPTER 5

Skin, Hair, and Nails

EQUIPMENT

- Centimeter ruler (flexible, clear)
- Flashlight with transilluminator
- Handheld magnifying lens or dermatoscope (optional)
- Wood's lamp (to view fluorescing lesions)

EXAMINATION

Technique	Findings

Skin

Perform overall inspection of entire body

In particular, check areas not usually exposed and intertriginous surfaces.	**EXPECTED:** Skin color differences among body areas and between sun-exposed and non–sun-exposed areas. **UNEXPECTED:** Lesions.

Inspect skin of each body area and mucous membranes

• *Color/uniformity* Inspect sclerae, conjunctivae, buccal mucosa, tongue, lips, nail beds, and palms.	**EXPECTED:** General uniformity— dark brown to light tan, with pink or yellow overtones. Sun-darkened areas. Darker skin around knees and elbows. Calloused areas yellow. Knuckles darker and palms/soles lighter in dark-skinned patients. Vascular flush areas pink or red, especially with anxiety or excitement.

Technique	Findings
Purpura—red-purple nonblanchable discoloration greater than 0.5 cm diameter. Cause: Intravascular defects, infection 	Spider angioma—red central body with radiating spiderlike legs that blanch with pressure to the central body. Cause: Liver disease, vitamin B deficiency, idiopathic 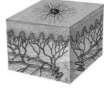
Petechiae—red-purple nonblanchable discoloration less than 0.5 cm diameter. Cause: Intravascular defects, infection	Venous star—bluish spider, linear or irregularly shaped; does not blanch with pressure. Cause: Increased pressure in superficial veins 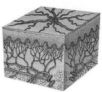
Ecchymoses—red-purple nonblanchable discoloration of variable size. Cause: Vascular wall destruction, trauma, vacculitis 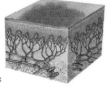	Telangiectasia—fine, irregular red line. Cause: Dilation of capillaries 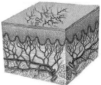
	Capillary hemangioma (nevus flammeus)—red irregular macular patches. Cause: Dilation of dermal capillaries 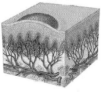

Cutaneous Color Changes

Color	Cause	Distribution	Select Conditions
Brown	Darkening of melanin pigment	Generalized	Pituitary, adrenal, liver disease Nevi, neurofibromatosis
White	Absence of pigmentation	Generalized Localized	Albinism Vitiligo
Red (erythema)	Increased cutaneous blood flow	Localized Generalized	Inflammation Fever, viral exanthems, urticaria
	Increased intravascular red blood cells	Generalized	Polycythemia

Continued

Cutaneous Color Changes—cont'd

Color	Cause	Distribution	Select Conditions
Yellow	Increased bile pigmentation (jaundice)	Generalized	Liver disease
	Increased carotene pigmentation	Generalized (except sclera)	Hypothyroidism, increased intake of vegetables containing carotene
	Decreased visibility of oxyhemoglobin	Generalized	Anemia, chronic renal disease
Blue	Increased unsaturated hemoglobin secondary to hypoxia	Lips, mouth, nail beds	Cardiovascular and pulmonary disease

Technique	Findings
	Pigmented nevi. Nonpigmented striae. Freckles. Birthmarks. **UNEXPECTED:** Dysplastic, precancerous, or cancerous nevi. Chloasma. Unpigmented skin. Generalized or localized color changes. Vascular skin lesions. Vascular changes.
• *Thickness*	**EXPECTED:** Thickness variations, with eyelids thinnest, areas of rubbing thickest. Calluses on hands and feet. **UNEXPECTED:** Atrophy. Hyperkeratosis. Corns.
• *Symmetry*	**EXPECTED:** Bilateral symmetry.
• *Hygiene*	**EXPECTED:** Clean.
Palpate skin.	
• *Moisture*	**EXPECTED:** Minimal perspiration or oiliness. Increased perspiration (associated with activity, environment, obesity, anxiety, excitement) noticeable on palms, scalp, forehead, axillae. **UNEXPECTED:** Damp intertriginous areas.
• *Temperature* Palpate with dorsal surface of hand or fingers.	**EXPECTED:** Cool to warm. Bilateral symmetry.

Technique	Findings
• *Texture*	**EXPECTED:** Smooth, soft, and even. Roughness resulting from heavy clothing, cold weather, or soap. **UNEXPECTED:** Extensive or widespread roughness.
• *Turgor and mobility* Gently pinch skin on forearm or in sternal area, and release.	**EXPECTED:** Resilience. **UNEXPECTED:** Failure of skin to return to place quickly.

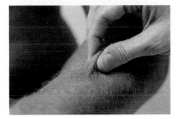

Inspect and palpate lesions

• *Size* Measure all dimensions. • *Shape* • *Color* Use Wood's lamp to distinguish fluorescing lesions. • *Blanching* • *Texture* Transilluminate to determine presence of fluid. • *Elevation/depression* • *Pedunculation* • *Exudate* Note color, odor, amount, and consistency of lesion. • *Configuration* Check lesion for annular, grouped, linear, arciform, or diffuse arrangement. • *Location/distribution* Check lesion for generalized/localized, body region, patterns, or discrete/confluent.	**UNEXPECTED:** See table on pp. 40-43.

SKIN, HAIR, AND NAILS

Primary Skin Lesions

Description	Examples

Macule

Flat, circumscribed area that is a change in skin color; <1 cm in diameter

Freckles, flat moles (nevi), petechiae, measles, scarlet fever

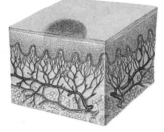

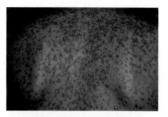

Measles. *(From Hockenberry and Wilson, 2007.)*

Papule

Elevated, firm, circumscribed area <1 cm in diameter

Wart (verruca), elevated moles, lichen planus

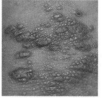

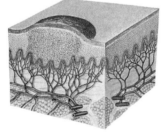

Lichen planus. *(From Weston et al, 1996.)*

Patch

Flat, nonpalpable, irregular-shaped macule >1 cm in diameter

Vitiligo, port-wine stains, mongolian spots, café-au-lait spots

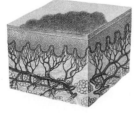

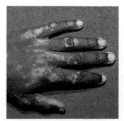

Vitiligo. *(From Weston et al, 1991.)*

Primary Skin Lesions—cont'd

Description	Examples

Plaque

Elevated, firm, and rough lesion with flat-top surface >1 cm in diameter

Psoriasis, seborrheic and actinic keratosis

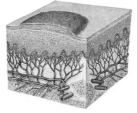

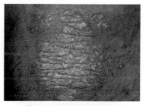

Plaque. *(From James et al, 2000.)*

Wheal

Elevated irregular shaped area of cutaneous edema; solid, transient; variable diameter

Insect bites, urticaria, allergic reaction

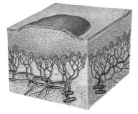

Wheal. *(From Farrar et al, 1992.)*

Nodule

Elevated, firm, circumscribed lesion; deeper in dermis than a papule; 1-2 cm in diameter

Erythema nodosum, lipomas

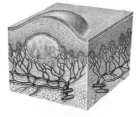

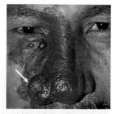

Hypertrophic nodule. *(From Goldman and Fitzpatrick, 1994.)*

Continued

SKIN, HAIR, AND NAILS

Primary Skin Lesions—cont'd

Description	Examples

Tumor

Elevated and solid lesion; may or may not be clearly demarcated; deeper in dermis; >2 cm in diameter

Neoplasms, benign tumor, lipoma, hemangioma

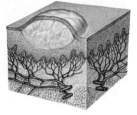

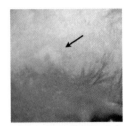

Hemangioma. *(From Weston et al, 1996.)*

Vesicle

Elevated, circumscribed, superficial, not into dermis; filled with serous fluid; <1 cm in diameter

Varicella (chickenpox), herpes zoster (shingles)

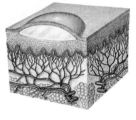

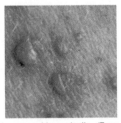

Vesicles caused by varicella. *(From Farrar et al, 1992.)*

Bulla

Vesicle >1 cm in diameter

Blister, pemphigus vulgaris

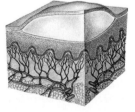

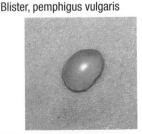

Blister. *(From White, 1994.)*

Primary Skin Lesions—cont'd

Description	Examples

Pustule

Elevated, superficial lesion; similar to a vesicle but filled with purulent fluid

Impetigo, acne

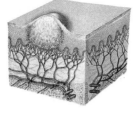

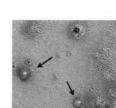

Acne. *(From Weston et al, 1996.)*

Cyst

Elevated, circumscribed, encapsulated lesion; in dermis or subcutaneous layer; filled with liquid or semisolid material

Sebaceous cyst, cystic acne

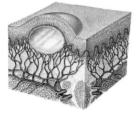

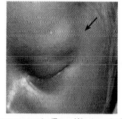

Sebaceous cyst. *(From Weston et al, 1996.)*

Telangiectasia

Fine, irregular red lines produced by capillary dilation

Telangiectasia in rosacea

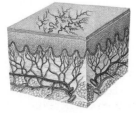

Telangiectasia. *(From Lemmi and Lemmi, 2000.)*

Technique	Findings
Hair	
Inspect hair over entire body	
• *Color*	**EXPECTED:** Light blond to black and gray, with alterations caused by rinses, dyes, and permanents.
• *Distribution/quantity*	**EXPECTED:** Hair present on scalp, lower face, neck, nares, ears, chest, axillae, back and shoulders, arms, legs, pubic area, and around nipples. Scalp hair loss in adult men, adrenal androgenic female-pattern alopecia in adult women. **UNEXPECTED:** Localized or generalized hair loss, inflammation, or scarring. Broken/absent hair shafts. Hirsutism in women.
Palpate for texture	**EXPECTED:** Coarse or fine, curly or straight, shiny, smooth, and resilient. Fine vellus covering body; coarse terminal hair on scalp, on pubis, on axillary areas, and in male beard. **UNEXPECTED:** Dryness and brittleness.
Nails	
Inspect nails	
• *Color*	**EXPECTED:** Variations of pink with varying opacity. Pigment deposits in persons with dark skin. White spots. **UNEXPECTED:** Yellow or green-black discoloration. Diffuse darkening. Pigment deposits in persons with light skin. Longitudinal red, brown, or white streaks or white bands. White, yellow, or green tinge. Blue nail beds. Blue-black discoloration.

Technique	Findings
• *Length/configuration/symmetry*	**EXPECTED:** Varying shape, smooth and flat/slightly convex, with edges smooth and rounded. **UNEXPECTED:** Jagged, broken, or bitten edges or cuticles. Peeling. Absence of nail.
• *Cleanliness*	**EXPECTED:** Clean and neat. **UNEXPECTED:** Unkempt.
• *Ridging and beading*	**EXPECTED:** Longitudinal ridging and beading. **UNEXPECTED:** Longitudinal ridging and grooving with lichen planus. Transverse grooving, rippling, and depressions. Pitting.

Palpate nail plate

• *Texture/firmness/thickness/uniformity*	**EXPECTED:** Hard and smooth with uniform thickness. **UNEXPECTED:** Thickening or thinning.
• *Adherence to nail bed* Gently squeeze between thumb and finger.	**EXPECTED:** Firmness. **UNEXPECTED:** Separation. Boggy nail base.

Measure nail base angle

Inspect fingers when patient places dorsal surfaces of fingertips together.	**EXPECTED:** 160-degree angle. **UNEXPECTED:** Clubbing.

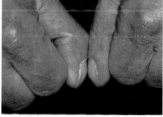

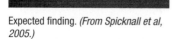

Expected finding. *(From Spicknall et al, 2005.)*

Clubbing. *(From Spicknall et al, 2005.)*

Inspect and palpate proximal and lateral nail folds

UNEXPECTED: Redness, swelling, pus, warts, cysts, tumors, and pain.

AIDS TO DIFFERENTIAL DIAGNOSIS

Subjective Data	Objective Data
Eczematous Dermatitis	
Itching may or may not be present; those with atopic dermatitis often report allergy history (allergic rhinitis, asthma).	Acute: erythematous, pruritic, weeping vesicles; subacute: erythema and scaling; chronic: thick, lichenified, pruritic plaques. Atopic dermatis: during childhood, lesions involve flexures, the nape, and the dorsal aspects of the limbs. In adolescence and adulthood, lichenified plaques affect the flexures, head, and neck.
Folliculitis	
Acute onset of papules and pustules associated with pruritus or mild discomfort; may have pain with deep folliculitis.	Primary lesion is a small pustule 1-2 cm in diameter that is located over a pilosebaceous orifice and may be perforated by a hair. Pustule may be surrounded by inflammation or nodular lesions. After the pustule ruptures, a crust forms.
Tinea (dermatophytosis)	
Pruritus.	Papular, pustular, vesicular, erythematous, or scaling lesions. Possible secondary bacterial infection. Hyphae on microscopic examination of skin scraping with KOH solution.
Rosacea	
Common triggers: sun, cold weather, sudden emotion, hot beverages, spicy foods, and alcohol	Telangiectasia, erythema, papules, and pustules particularly in the central area of the face; rhinophyma may occur
Herpes Zoster (Shingles)	
Pain, itching, or burning usually precedes eruption by 4-5 days	Red, swollen plaques or vesicles along a single dermatome

Subjective Data	Objective Data
Basal Cell Carcinoma Persistent sore or lesions that have not healed; crusting; itching.	Shiny nodule that is pearly or translucent; may be pink, red, white, tan, black, or brown growth with a slightly elevated rolled border and a crusted indentation in the center.
Squamous Cell Carcinoma Persistent sore or lesion that has not healed or that has grown in size; crusting and/or bleeding.	Elevated growth with a central depression, wartlike growth; scaly red patch with irregular borders; open sore.
Malignant Melanoma New mole or preexisting mole that has changed or is changing; history of melanoma, dysplastic or atypical nevi; family history of melanoma.	Characteristic asymmetry, irregular borders, variegated colors, and is growing or >6 mm (see ABCDs of Melanoma on pp. 49-50).
Hirsutism Growth of terminal hair in women in the male distribution pattern on the face, body, and pubic areas.	Presence of thick, dark terminal hairs in androgen-sensitive sites: face, chest, areola, external genitalia, upper and lower back, buttock, inner thigh, linea.
Paronychia Acute: history of nail trauma or manipulation; acute onset. Chronic: history of repeated exposure to moisture, e.g., through hand-washing. Evolves slowly initially with tenderness and mild swelling.	Redness, swelling, tenderness at lateral and proximal nail folds. Possible purulent drainage under cuticle. Acute or chronic (with nail rippling).
Onychomycosis Yellow, crumbling nail.	Distal nail plate turns yellow or white as hyperkeratotic debris accumulates, causing the nail to separate from the nail bed. Redness and swelling where nail pierces the lateral nail fold and grows into the dermis.

SKIN, HAIR, AND NAILS

PEDIATRIC VARIATIONS

EXAMINATION

Technique	Findings

Skin

Inspect hands and feet of newborns for skin creases

EXPECTED: Number of creases is indication of maturity of newborn; the older the gestational age, the more creases.

UNEXPECTED: Single transverse crease across palm frequently seen in infants with Down syndrome.

AIDS TO DIFFERENTIAL DIAGNOSIS

Subjective Data	Objective Data

Seborrheic Dermatitis

Thick greasy scalp scales or body rash.	Thick, yellow, adherent crusted scalp, ear, or neck lesions.

Impetigo

Lesion, typically on the face, that itches and burns.	Honey-colored crusted or ruptured vesicles.

Miliaria ("prickly heat")

Parent reports rash noted while undressing infant.	Irregular, red, macular rash on covered areas.

Chickenpox (varicella)

Fever, headache, sore throat, malaise.	Pruritic maculopapular skin eruption that becomes vesicular in a matter of hours.

German measles (rubella)

Fever, coryza, sore throat, cough.	Koplik spots on buccal mucosa; generalized light pink to red maculopapular rash.

SAMPLE DOCUMENTATION

Objective

Skin: Dark pink maculopapular lesions on face, torso, extremities; large urticarial wheal on right cheek. No excoriation or secondary infection. Turgor resilient. Skin uniformly warm and dry. No edema.

Hair: Curly, black, thick with female distribution pattern. Texture coarse.

Nails: Opaque, short, well-groomed, uniform, and without deformities. Nail bed pink. Nail base angle 160 degrees. No redness, exudates, or swelling in surrounding folds and no tenderness to palpation.

The ABCDs of Melanoma

Characteristics that should alert you to the possibility of malignant melanoma:

A Asymmetry of lesion: Half of a mole or birthmark does not match the other.

B Borders: Edges are irregular, ragged, notched, or blurred. Pigment may be streaming from the border.

C Color: The color is not the same all over and may have differing shades of brown or black, sometimes with patches of red, white, or blue.

D Diameter: The diameter is larger than 6 mm (about the size of a pencil eraser) or is growing larger.

SKIN, HAIR, AND NAILS

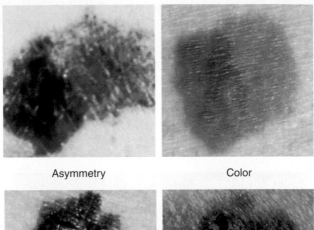

Asymmetry   Color

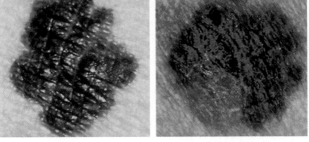

Border   Diameter

CHAPTER 6

Lymphatic System

EQUIPMENT

- Centimeter ruler
- Skin-marking pencil

EXAMINATION

The lymphatic system is examined by inspection and palpation, region by region, during the examination of other body systems, and by palpating the spleen. If enlarged nodes are found, inspect regions drained by nodes for infection or malignancy and examine other regions for enlargement.

Lymph Nodes Most Accessible to Inspection and Palpation

The more superficial the node, the more accessible it is to your palpation.

"Necklace" of Nodes
Parotid and retropharyngeal (tonsillar)
Submandibular
Submental
Sublingual (facial)
Superficial anterior cervical
Superficial posterior cervical

Preauricular and postauricular
Occipital
Supraclavicular

Arms
Axillary
Epitrochlear (cubital)

Legs
Superficial superior inguinal
Superficial inferior inguinal
Occasionally, popliteal

Technique	Findings
Head and Neck	
Inspect for visible nodes	
Ask if patient is aware of any lumps.	**UNEXPECTED:** Edema, erythema, red streaks, or lesions.

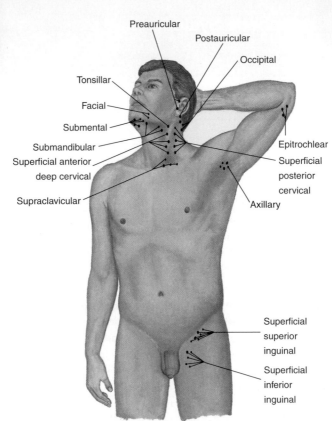

G. J. Wassilchenko

Palpate superficial nodes; note size, consistency, mobility, tenderness, warmth

Bend patient's head slightly forward or to side. Palpate gently with pads of second, third, fourth fingers.

- *Occipital nodes at base of skull*
- *Postauricular nodes over mastoid process*
- *Preauricular nodes in front of ears*
- *Parotid and retropharyngeal nodes at angle of mandible*
- *Submandibular nodes between angle and tip of mandible*
- *Submental nodes behind tip of mandible*

EXPECTED: Nodes not palpable.
UNEXPECTED: Enlarged, tender, red or discolored, fixed, matted, inflamed, or warm nodes; increased vascularity.

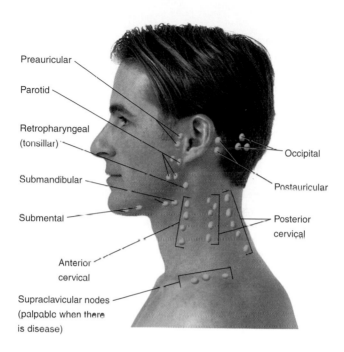

Preauricular

Parotid

Retropharyngeal
(tonsillar)

Submandibular

Submental

Anterior
cervical

Supraclavicular nodes
(palpable when there
is disease)

Occipital

Postauricular

Posterior
cervical

Neck

- *Superficial cervical nodes at sternocleidomastoid*
- *Posterior cervical nodes along anterior border of trapezius*
- *Deep cervical nodes along anterior border of trapezius*
- *Supraclavicular areas*
  Hook fingers over clavicle and rotate over supraclavicular fossa while patient turns head toward same side and raises shoulder.

EXPECTED: Nodes not palpable.
UNEXPECTED: Enlarged, tender, red or discolored, fixed, matted, inflamed, or warm nodes; increased vascularity.

UNEXPECTED: Detection of Virchow nodes.
NOTE: A palpable supraclavicular node should always make you suspect the probability of a malignancy.

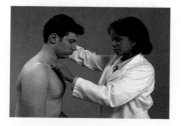

Axillae

Inspect for visible nodes

Ask if patient is aware of any lumps.

UNEXPECTED: Edema, erythema, red streaks, or lesions.

Palpate superficial nodes for size, consistency, mobility, tenderness, warmth

Using firm, deliberate, gentle touch, rotate fingertips and palm.
Attempt to glide fingers beneath nodes.

Axillary nodes

Support patient's forearm and bring palm of examining hand flat into axilla. With palmar surface of fingers, reach deep into hollow, pushing firmly upward, then bring fingers down, rotating your fingers and gently rolling soft tissue against chest wall and axilla. Explore apex, medial, lateral aspects along rib cage; lateral aspects along upper surface of arm; and anterior and posterior walls of axilla. Repeat mirror image of this maneuver for the other axilla.

EXPECTED: Nodes not palpable.
UNEXPECTED: Enlarged, tender, red or discolored, fixed, matted, inflamed, or warm nodes; increased vascularity.

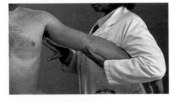

Other Lymph Nodes

Inspect visible nodes

Ask if patient is aware of any lumps.

UNEXPECTED: Edema, erythema, red streaks, or lesions.

Palpate superficial nodes for size, consistency, mobility, tenderness, warmth

Systematically palpate other areas, moving hand in circular fashion, probing without pressing hard.

EXPECTED: Nodes not palpable.
UNEXPECTED: Enlarged, tender, red or discolored, fixed, matted, inflamed, or warm nodes; increased vascularity.

- *Epitrochlear nodes*
  Support elbow in one hand while exploring with other. Palpate that groove between the triceps and biceps muscle with your fingers using a circular motion.

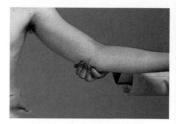

- *Inguinal area*
  Have patient lie supine with knee slightly flexed. The superior superficial inguinal (femoral) nodes are close to the surface over the inguinal canals. The inferior superficial inguinal nodes lie deeper in the groin.

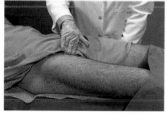 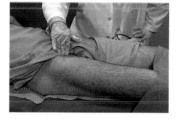

- *Popliteal nodes*
  Relax the posterior popliteal fossa by flexing the knee. Wrap your hand around the knee and palpate the fossa with your fingers.

AIDS TO DIFFERENTIAL DIAGNOSIS

Subjective Data	Objective Data
Acute Lymphangitis	
Pain, malaise, illness, possibly fever.	Red streak (tracing of fine lines) may follow course of lymphatic collecting duct. Inflamed area indurated and palpable to gentle touch. Related infection possible distally, particularly interdigitally.

Non-Hodgkin Lymphoma

Painless enlarged lymph node(s); fever, weight loss, night sweats, abdominal pain or fullness.

Nodes may be localized in the posterior cervical triangle or may become matted, crossing into the anterior triangle nodes; usually well-defined and solid.

Hodgkin Lymphoma

Painless progressive enlargement of cervical lymph nodes. Generally asymmetric.

Nodes sometimes matted and generally very firm, almost rubbery.

Epstein-Barr Virus; Mononucleosis

Pharyngitis, fever, fatigue, malaise.

Frequently splenomegaly and/or rash. Palpable nodes generalized but more commonly in anterior and posterior cervical chains. Nodes vary in firmness, are generally discrete, are occasionally tender.

Roseola Infantum (human herpes virus-6)

Fever: usually high grade and persistent over 3-4 days; sometimes associated with a mild respiratory illness

Discrete and nontender nodes in the occipital and postauricular chains.

Herpes Simplex

Burning, itching lesions; enlarged lymph nodes.

Discrete labial and gingival ulcers, high fever, enlargement of anterior cervical and submandibular nodes. Nodes tend to be firm, quite discrete, movable, tender.

Human Immunodeficiency Virus/Acquired Immunodeficiency Syndrome (HIV/AIDS)

Severe fatigue, malaise, weakness, persistent diarrhea; arthralgias.

Lymphadenopathy, fever, unexplained weight loss.

Terms

Conditions

Lymphadenopathy (adenopathy)—enlarged lymph node(s)

Lymphadenitis—inflamed and enlarged lymph node(s)

Lymphangitis—inflammation of the lymphatics that drain an area of infection; tender erythematous streaks extend proximally from the infected area; regional nodes may also be tender

Lymphedema—edematous swelling caused by excess accumulation of lymph fluid in tissues caused by inadequate lymph drainage

Lymphangioma—congenital malformation of dilated lymphatics

Nodes

Shotty—small nontender nodes that feel like BBs or buckshot under the skin

Fluctuant—wavelike motion that is felt when the node is palpated

Matted—group of nodes that feel connected and seem to move as a unit

Some Conditions That Simulate Lymph Node Enlargement

Lymphangioma

Hemangioma (tends to feel spongy; appears reddish blue, depending on size and extent of angiomatous involvement)

Branchial cleft cyst (sometimes accompanied by tiny orifice in neck on line extending to ear)

Thyroglossal duct cyst

Laryngocele

Esophageal diverticulum

Thyroid goiter

Graves disease

Hashimoto thyroiditis

Parotid swelling (e.g., from mumps or tumor)

LYMPHATIC SYSTEM

PEDIATRIC VARIATIONS

EXAMINATION

Technique	Findings
Head and Neck	
Palpate superficial nodes	
• Occipital nodes at base of skull	**EXPECTED:** In children, small, firm, discrete, nontender, nonmovable nodes in occipital, postauricular chains.
• Postauricular nodes over mastoid process	
Other Lymph Nodes	
Palpate superficial nodes	
• Inguinal and popliteal areas	**EXPECTED:** In children, small, firm, discrete nodes; nontender, movable in inguinal chain.

SAMPLE DOCUMENTATION

Subjective. A 25-year-old woman reports difficulty swallowing and sore throat for 3 days, now subsiding. Fever to 38° C (100.5° F) for 2 days. Has been using acetaminophen and throat lozenges for pain relief.

Objective. No visible enlargement of lymph nodes in any area. Enlarged node (2 cm in diameter) palpated in left posterior cervical triangle; firm, nontender, movable, no overlying warmth, erythema, or edema. A few shotty nodes palpated in posterior cervical triangles bilaterally and in femoral chains bilaterally.

CHAPTER 7

Head and Neck

EQUIPMENT

- Tape measure
- Cup of water
- Stethoscope
- Transilluminator

EXAMINATION

Ask patient to sit.

Technique	Findings
Head and Face	
Observe head position	**EXPECTED:** Upright, midline, still. **UNEXPECTED:** Tilted, horizontal jerking or bobbing, tics, nodding.
Inspect facial features	
• *Shape* Observe eyelids, eyebrows, palpebral fissures, nasolabial folds, mouth at rest, during movement, with expression.	**EXPECTED:** Variations according to race, sex, age, body build. **UNEXPECTED:** Change in shape. Unusual features: edema, puffiness, coarsened features, prominent eyes, hirsutism, lack of expression, excessive perspiration, pallor, or pigmentation variations.
• *Symmetry* Note if asymmetry affects all features of one side or a portion of face.	**EXPECTED:** Slight asymmetry. **UNEXPECTED:** Facial nerve weakness or paralysis, or problem with peripheral trigeminal nerve.
Inspect skull and scalp	
• *Size/shape/symmetry* • *Scalp condition* • *Systematically part hair from frontal to occipital region.*	**EXPECTED:** Symmetric. **UNEXPECTED:** Lesions, scabs, tenderness, parasites, nits, scaliness. **EXPECTED:** Bitemporal recession or balding over crown in men.
• *Hair pattern* Pay special attention to areas behind ears, at hairline, at crown.	**UNEXPECTED:** Random areas of alopecia or alopecia totalis.

Palpate head and scalp

- *Symmetry*
  Palpate in gentle, rotary
  motion from front to back.

EXPECTED: Symmetric and smooth with bones indistinguishable. Ridge of sagittal fissure occasionally palpable.
UNEXPECTED: Indentations or depressions.

Palpate hair

- *Texture/color distribution*

EXPECTED: Smooth, symmetrically distributed.
UNEXPECTED: Splitting or cracked ends. Coarse, dry, or brittle. Fine and silky.

Palpate temporal arteries
Note course of arteries.

UNEXPECTED: Thickening, hardness, or tenderness.

Auscultate temporal arteries and over skull and eyes

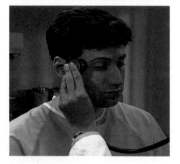

EXPECTED: No bruits.

Inspect salivary glands

- *Symmetry/size*
  Palpate if asymmetry noted.
  Have patient open mouth
  and press on salivary duct to
  attempt to express material.

UNEXPECTED: Asymmetry or enlargement. Tenderness. Discrete nodule.

Neck

Inspect neck

- *Symmetry*
  Inspect in usual position, in
  slight hyperextension, and
  during swallowing. Look for
  landmarks of anterior and
  posterior triangles.

EXPECTED: Bilateral symmetry of sternocleidomastoid and trapezius muscles.
UNEXPECTED: Asymmetry, torticollis webbing, excessive posterior skinfolds, unusually short

- *Trachea*
  Inspect in usual position, in slight hyperextension, and while patient swallows.

neck, distention of jugular vein; prominence of carotid arteries, or edema.
EXPECTED: Midline placement.
UNEXPECTED: Masses.

Evaluate range of motion

Have patient flex, extend, rotate, laterally turn head and neck.

EXPECTED: Smooth.
UNEXPECTED: Pain, dizziness, or limitation of motion.

Palpate neck

- *Trachea*
  Place thumb on each side of trachea in lower portion of neck, and compare space between trachea and sternocleidomastoid on each side.

EXPECTED: Midline position.
UNEXPECTED: Deviation to right or left.

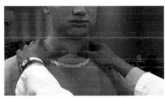

- *Hyoid bone/thyroid and cricoid cartilages*
  Have patient swallow.
- *Cartilaginous rings of trachea*
  Have patient swallow.
- *Tracheal tug*
  With neck extended, palpate for movement with index finger and thumb on each side of trachea below thyroid isthmus.

EXPECTED: Smooth. Moves during swallowing.
UNEXPECTED: Tender.
EXPECTED: Distinct.
UNEXPECTED: Tender.
UNEXPECTED: Tug synchronous with pulse.

Palpate lymph nodes

- *Size/consistency, mobility/condition*

UNEXPECTED: Enlarged, matted, tender, fixed, warm.

HEAD AND NECK

Palpate thyroid gland

- *Symmetry*
  Observe from frontal and lateral positions while patient hyperextends neck. Then observe as patient sips water while neck is hyperextended.

UNEXPECTED: Asymmetry. Enlarged and visible thyroid gland.

- *Size/shape/configuration/ consistency*
  Stand either facing or behind patient. Have patient hold head slightly forward and tipped toward side being examined. Lightly palpate isthmus and lateral lobes. Give water to patient to facilitate swallowing.

  From the front, examine the left lobe by sitting on the left side of the patient and pressing the trachea to the left with the left thumb. Place the first three fingers in the thyroid bed just medial to the sternocleidomastoid. Keep your fingers still while the patient again swallows, thereby moving the gland beneath your fingers.

  Repeat on the right side.

  If gland is enlarged, auscultate for vascular sounds with stethoscope bell.

EXPECTED: Lobes small and smooth. Gland rises freely with swallowing. Right lobe as much as 25% larger than left. Tissue firm and pliable.
UNEXPECTED: Enlarged, tender nodules (smooth or irregular, soft or hard); coarse tissue; gritty sensation.
UNEXPECTED: Bruit.

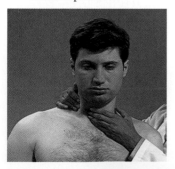

AIDS TO DIFFERENTIAL DIAGNOSIS

Subjective Data	Objective Data

Myxedema

Cognitive impairment, slowed mentation, poor concentration, decreased short-term memory, social withdrawal, psychomotor retardation, depressed mood, and apathy.

Dull, puffy, yellow skin. Coarse, sparse hair. Temporal loss of eyebrows. Periorbital edema. Prominent tongue. Hypothyroidism (see table on p. 66).

Graves Disease

Symptoms of hyperthyroidism, palpitations, heat intolerance, weight loss, fatigue, increased appetite, tachycardia.

Diffuse thyroid enlargement, hyperthyroidism. Various pathologic conditions—ophthalmologic (prominent eyes, lid retraction, staring or startled expression), dermatologic (fine and moist skin, fine hair), musculoskeletal (muscle weakness), cardiac (tachycardia) (see table on p. 66).

HEAD AND NECK

Headaches

Headaches are one of the most common concerns and probably one of the most self-medicated. They are not always benign. A history of insistent headache that is severe and recurrent must always be given attention. Sometimes the underlying cause is life-threatening, such as a brain tumor. Sometimes it affects daily activities. The patient's history is fully as important as the physical examination in getting at the root of a headache. Various kinds of headaches can be compared as follows:

Charac-teristic	Classic Migraine	Medication Rebound	Cluster	Hyperten-sive	Muscular Tension	Temporal Arteritis	Space-Occupying Lesion
Age at onset	Childhood		Adulthood	Adulthood	Adulthood	Older adult-hood	Any
Location	Unilateral or generalized	Holocranial or diffuse	Unilateral	Bilateral or occipital	Unilateral or bilateral	Unilateral or bilateral	Localized
Duration	Hours to days	Hours	½ to 2 hours	Hours	Hours to days	Hours to days	Rapidly increasing frequency
Time of onset	Morning or night	Predictably begins within hours to days of the last dose of the medication	Night	Morning	Anytime, commonly in afternoon or evening	Anytime	Awakening from sleep
Quality of pain	Pulsating or throbbing	Dull or throbbing	Intense burning, boring, searing, knifelike	Throbbing	Bandlike, constricting	Throbbing	

Prodromal event	Vague neurologic changes, personality change, fluid retention, appetite loss Well-defined neurologic event, scotoma, aphasia, hemianopsia, aura	Daily analgesic use	None	Personality changes sleep disturbances	None	None	Aggravated by coughing or bending forward
Precipitating event	Menstrual period, missing meals, birth control pills, letdown after stress	Abrupt discontinuation of analgesics	Alcohol consumption	None	Stress, anger, bruxism	None	Develops in temporal relation to the neoplasm
Frequency	Twice a week	Gradual increase in headache frequency to daily	Several times nightly for several nights, then none	Daily	Daily	Daily	Progressive
Sex predilection	Females	Females	Males	Equal	Equal	Equal	Equal
Other symptoms	Nausea, vomiting	Alternate or preventive medications fail to control the headache	Increased lacrimation, nasal discharge	Generally remits as day progresses	None	None	Vomiting, confusion, abnormal neurologic findings, gait abnormality, papilledema, nystagmus

HEAD AND NECK

Hyperthyroidism versus Hypothyroidism

System or Structure Affected	Hyperthyroidism	Hypothyroidism
Constitutional		
Temperature preference	Cool climate	Warm climate
Weight	Loss	Gain
Emotional state	Nervous, easily irritated, highly energetic	Lethargic, complacent, uninterested
Hair	Fine, with hair loss; failure to hold permanent wave	Coarse, with tendency to break
Skin	Warm, fine, hyperpigmentation at pressure points	Coarse, scaling, dry
Fingernails	Thin, with tendency to break; may show onycholysis	Thick
Eyes	Bilateral or unilateral proptosis, lid retraction, double vision	Puffiness in periorbital region
Neck	Goiter, change in shirt neck size, pain over thyroid	No goiter
Cardiac	Tachycardia, dysrhythmia, palpitations	No change noted
Gastrointestinal	Increased frequency of bowel movements; diarrhea rare	Constipation
Menstrual	Scant flow, amenorrhea	Menorrhagia
Neuromuscular	Increasing weakness, especially of proximal muscles	Lethargic, but good muscular strength

PEDIATRIC VARIATIONS

EXAMINATION

Technique	Findings

Head and Face

Palpate head and scalp

- *Symmetry*
  In infants, transilluminate skull

EXPECTED: An infant's head circumference is 2 cm greater than chest circumference up to the age of 2 yr.

UNEXPECTED: Ring of light greater than 2 cm with transillumination.

- *Skull condition*

  EXPECTED: In infants, posterior fontanel closed at 2 mo; anterior fontanel closed at 12-15 mo.
  UNEXPECTED: Tenderness or depressions; sunken areas; swelling, bulging, or depressed fontanels.

- *Scalp*

  EXPECTED: Free movement.
  UNEXPECTED: Fixation of scalp, bulging either on one side or crossing midline of scalp.

Percuss skull

EXPECTED: Macewen sign, percussion near junction of frontal, temporal, and parietal bones producing a stronger resonant sound, is physiologic when fontanels are open.
UNEXPECTED: Macewen sign may indicate hydrocephalus, a brain abscess is present, or increased intracranial pressure after fontanel closure.

Auscultate temporal arteries and over skull and eyes

EXPECTED: Bruits are common in children up to age 5 yr.

Neck

Palpate thyroid gland

- *Symmetry*

  EXPECTED: In children, thyroid gland may be palpable.
  UNEXPECTED: Tenderness.

SAMPLE DOCUMENTATION

Head. Held erect and midline. Skull normocephalic, symmetric, smooth without deformities. Facial features symmetric. Salivary glands not inflamed or tender. Temporal artery pulsations visible bilaterally, soft and nontender to palpation. No bruits.

Neck. Trachea midline. No jugular venous distention or carotid artery prominence. Thyroid palpable, firm, smooth, not enlarged. Thyroid and cartilages move with swallowing. No nodules or tenderness. No bruits. Full range of motion of neck without discomfort.

CHAPTER 8

Eyes

EQUIPMENT

- Snellen chart or Lea cards, Landolt C or HOTV chart
- Eye cover, gauze, or opaque card
- Rosenbaum or Jaeger near-vision card
- Penlight
- Cotton wisp
- Ophthalmoscope

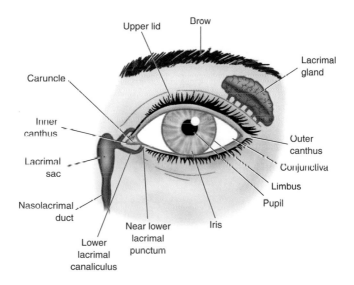

EXAMINATION

Ask patient to sit or stand.

EYES

Technique	Findings

Visual Testing

Measure visual acuity in each eye separately

- *Distance vision*
  Use Snellen chart, Landolt C, or HOTV chart. If testing with and without corrective lenses, test without lenses first and record readings separately.

  EXPECTED: Vision 20/20 with or without lenses with near and far vision in each eye.
  UNEXPECTED: Myopia, amblyopia, or presbyopia.

- *Near vision*
  Use near-vision card.

  EXPECTED: Vision 20/20.
  UNEXPECTED: Limited fields of vision temporally, 50 degrees superiorly, 70 degrees inferiorly.

- *Peripheral vision*
  Test nasal, temporal, superior, inferior fields by moving your finger into field from outside.

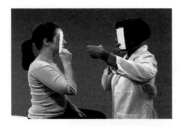

External Examination

Inspect eyebrows

- *Size/extension*

  EXPECTED: Unusually thin if plucked.
  UNEXPECTED: Ending short of temporal canthus.

- *Hair texture*

  UNEXPECTED: Coarse.

Inspect orbital area

  UNEXPECTED: Edema, puffiness not related to aging, or sagging tissue below orbit. Xanthelasma.

Inspect eyelids

- *Eyelid position*

  UNEXPECTED: Ectropion or entropion.

- *Ability to open wide and close completely*
  Examine with eyes lightly closed, closed tightly, open wide.

- *Eyelid margin*

- *Eyelashes*

Palpate eyelids

Palpate eye

Pull down lower lids and inspect conjunctivae and sclerae

- *Color*
  Inspect upper tarsal conjunctivae only if presence of foreign body is suspected.

- *Appearance*

Inspect lacrimal gland region

- *Lacrimal gland puncta*
  Palpate lower orbital rim near inner canthus. If temporal aspect of upper lid feels full, evert lid and inspect gland.

Test corneal sensitivity
Touch wisp of cotton to cornea.

Inspect external eyes

- *Corneal clarity*
  Shine light tangentially on cornea.

EXPECTED: Superior eyelid covering a portion of iris when open.
UNEXPECTED: Fasciculations when lightly closed. Ptosis. Lagophthalmos.

UNEXPECTED: Flakiness, redness, or swelling. Hordeola.
EXPECTED: Present on both lids. Turned outward.

UNEXPECTED: Nodules.

EXPECTED: Can be gently pushed into orbit without discomfort.
UNEXPECTED: Firm and resists palpation.

EXPECTED: Conjunctivae clear and inapparent. Sclerae white and visible above irides only when eyelids are wide open.
UNEXPECTED: Conjunctivae with erythema. Sclerae yellow or green. Sclerae with dark, rust-colored pigment anterior to insertion of medial rectus muscle.

UNEXPECTED: Exudate. Pterygium. Corneal arcus senilis or opacities.

EXPECTED: Slight elevations with central depression on both upper and lower lid margins.
UNEXPECTED: Enlarged glands. Dry eyes.

EXPECTED: Bilateral blink reflex.

UNEXPECTED: Blood vessels present.

EYES

- *Irides*

  EXPECTED: Clearly visible pattern. Similar color.

- *Pupillary size/shape*

  EXPECTED: Round, regular, equal in size.

  UNEXPECTED: Miosis, mydriasis, anisocoria, or coloboma.

- *Pupillary response to light*

  EXPECTED: Constricting with consensual response of opposite pupil.

- *Pupillary accommodation*

  EXPECTED: Constricting when pupils focus on near object or dilating when focus changes from near to distant object.

- *Afferent pupillary testing*

  EXPECTED: The pupil toward which the light is moving dilates and then constricts as the light shines onto it.

  UNEXPECTED: The pupil continues to dilate when the light shines into it.

Extraocular Eye Muscles
Evaluate muscle balance and movement of eyes

- *Six cardinal fields of gaze*
  Hold patient's chin and ask patient to watch finger or penlight.

  EXPECTED: A few horizontal nystagmic beats. Smooth, full, coordinated movement of eyes.

  UNEXPECTED: Sustained or jerking nystagmus. Exposure of sclera from lid lag. Inability of eye to move in all directions.

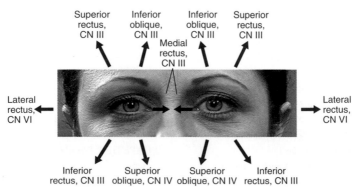

Superior rectus, CN III   Inferior oblique, CN III   Inferior oblique, CN III   Superior rectus, CN III

Medial rectus, CN III

Lateral rectus, CN VI   Lateral rectus, CN VI

Inferior rectus, CN III   Superior oblique, CN IV   Superior oblique, CN IV   Inferior rectus, CN III

- *Corneal light reflex*
  Direct light at nasal bridge
      from 30 cm (12 inches). Have
      patient look at nearby object.

EXPECTED: Light reflected
symmetrically from both eyes.

- *Cover-uncover test*
  Perform if imbalance found
      with corneal light reflex test.
      Have patient stare ahead at
      near, fixed object. Cover one
      eye and observe other; remove
      cover and observe uncovered eye.
      Repeat with other eye.

UNEXPECTED: Movement of
covered or uncovered eye.

Ophthalmoscopic Examination
Inspect internal eye

- *Lens clarity*

UNEXPECTED: Cloudiness or
opacity. Shallow chamber. If
observed, avoid mydriatics

- *Anterior chamber*
  Shine focused light tangentially
      at limbus. Note illumination
      of iris nasally.

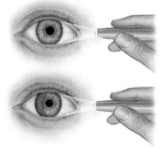

- *Use ophthalmoscope*
  With patient looking at distant
      object, direct light at pupil from
      about 30 cm (12 inches). Move
      toward patient, observing:
  - *Red reflex*

UNEXPECTED: Opacities.

EYES

• *Fundus*

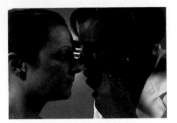

EXPECTED: Yellow or pink background, depending on race. Possible crescents or dots of pigment at disc margin, usually temporally.
UNEXPECTED: Discrete areas of pigmentation away from disc. Lesions. Drusen bodies. Hemorrhages.

• *Blood vessel characteristics*
  Follow blood vessels distally in each quadrant, noting crossings of arterioles and venules.

EXPECTED: Possible venous pulsations (should be documented). Arteriole/venule ratio 3:5 or 2:3.
UNEXPECTED: Nicking, tortuosity.

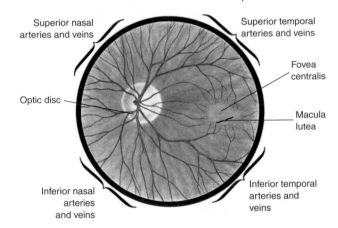

Superior nasal arteries and veins

Superior temporal arteries and veins

Fovea centralis

Optic disc

Macula lutea

Inferior nasal arteries and veins

Inferior temporal arteries and veins

• *Disc characteristics*

EXPECTED: Yellow to creamy pink, varying by race. Sharp, well-defined margin, especially in temporal region; 1.5-mm diameter.
UNEXPECTED: Myelinated nerve fibers. Papilledema. Glaucomatous cupping.

• *Macula densa characteristics*
  Ask patient to look directly at light.

EXPECTED: Yellow dot surrounded by deep pink.

AIDS TO DIFFERENTIAL DIAGNOSIS

Subjective Data	Objective Data

Strabismus (paralytic and nonparalytic)

Eyes cannot focus simultaneously. Can focus separately in nonparalytic type.

Eye movement on the cover-uncover test, strabismic eye will fixate on the object after the "straight" eye is covered.

Episcleritis

Acute onset of mild to moderate discomfort or photophobia. Painless injection and/or watery discharge.

Injection of the bulbar conjunctiva purplish elevation of a few millimeters.

Cataracts

Cloudy or blurry vision, faded colors; halo may appear around lights.

Opacity of lens, generally central, occasionally peripheral.

Diabetic Retinopathy (background or nonproliferative)

Initially asymptomatic. Blurred vision, distortion, or visual acuity loss in more advanced stages.

Dot hemorrhages, microaneurysms, hard exudates.

Diabetic Retinopathy (proliferative)

Generally asymptomatic, floaters, blurred vision, or progressive visual acuity loss in advanced stages.

New vessel formation; extension out of the retina, hemorrhage.

PEDIATRIC VARIATIONS

EXAMINATION

Technique	Findings

Visual Testing

Measure visual acuity

• *Distance vision*
Visual acuity is tested, when child is cooperative, with Lea cards, Landolt C, or HOTV chart, usually at about 3 years of age.

EXPECTED: Infants should be able to focus on and track a face or light through 60 degrees.
Age 3-5 years: 20/40 or better. Age 6: 20/30 or better.

Extraocular Eye Muscles

Evaluate muscle balance and movement of eyes

Evaluation of six cardinal fields of gaze is performed as with adults. You may, however, need to hold child's head still.

SAMPLE DOCUMENTATION

Eyes. Near vision 20/40 in each eye uncorrected, corrected to 20/20 with glasses. Distant vision 20/20 by Snellen. Visual fields full by confrontation. Extraocular movements intact and full, no nystagmus. Corneal light reflex equal.

Lids and globes symmetric. No ptosis. Eyebrows full, no edema or lesions evident.

Conjunctivae pink, sclerae white. No discharge evident. Cornea clear, corneal reflex intact. Irides brown; pupils equal, round, reactive to light and accommodation.

Ophthalmoscopic examination reveals red reflex. Discs cream colored, borders well defined with temporal pigmentation in both eyes. No venous pulsations evident at disc. Arteriole/venule ratio 3:5; no nicking or crossing changes, hemorrhages, or exudates noted. Maculae are yellow in each eye.

EYES

CHAPTER 9

Ears, Nose, and Throat

EQUIPMENT

- Otoscope with pneumatic attachment
- Tuning fork (512-1024 Hz)
- Nasal speculum
- Tongue blades
- Gloves
- Gauze
- Penlight, sinus transilluminator, or light from otoscope

EXAMINATION

Have patient sit.

Technique	Findings

Ears

Inspect auricles and mastoid area
Examine lateral and medial surfaces and surrounding tissue.

Auricle landmarks

- *Size/shape/symmetry*

EXPECTED: Familial variations. Auricles of equal size and similar appearance. Darwin tubercle.
UNEXPECTED: Unequal size or configuration. Cauliflower ear and other deformities.

- *Lesions*

  UNEXPECTED: Moles, cysts or other lesions, nodules, or tophi.

- *Color*

  EXPECTED: Same color as facial skin.
  UNEXPECTED: Blueness, pallor, or excessive redness.

- *Position*
  Draw imaginary line between inner canthus and most prominent protuberance of occiput. Draw imaginary line perpendicular to first line and anterior to auricle.

  EXPECTED: Top of auricle touching or above horizontal line. Auricle is in vertical position.
  UNEXPECTED: Auricle positioned below line (low-set); unequal alignment. Lateral posterior angle greater than 10 degrees.

- *Preauricular area*

  EXPECTED: Preauricular pits, skin tags, or smooth skin.
  UNEXPECTED: Openings in preauricular area, discharge.

- *External auditory canal*

  EXPECTED: No discharge, no odor; canal walls pink.
  UNEXPECTED: Serous, bloody, or purulent discharge; foul smell.

Palpate auricles and mastoid area

EXPECTED: Firm and mobile, readily recoils from folded position; no tenderness in postauricular or mastoid area.
UNEXPECTED: Tenderness, swelling, nodules. Pain when pulling on lobule.

Inspect auditory canal with otoscope
Slowly insert the otoscope speculum to a depth of 1 to 1½ cm (½ inch) inspecting the auditory canal from the meatus to the tympanic membrane.

EXPECTED: Minimal cerumen in varying color and texture. Uniformly pink canal. Hairs in outer third of canal.
UNEXPECTED: Cerumen obscures tympanic membrane, odor, lesions, discharge, scaling, excessive redness, foreign body.

Inspect tympanic membrane
- *Landmarks*
  Vary light direction to observe entire membrane and annulus.

  EXPECTED: Visible landmarks (umbo, handle of malleus, light reflex).
  UNEXPECTED: Perforations, landmarks not visible.

- *Color*

  EXPECTED: Translucent, pearly gray.

  UNEXPECTED: Amber, yellow, blue, deep red, chalky white, dull, white flecks, or dense white plaques; air bubbles or fluid level.

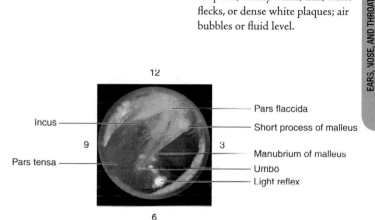

Tympanic membrane. *(From Barkauskas et al, 2001.)*

- *Contour*

  EXPECTED: Slightly conical with concavity at umbo.

  UNEXPECTED: Bulging (more conical, usually with loss of bony landmarks and distorted light reflex) or retracted (more concave, usually with accentuated bony landmarks and distorted light reflex).

- *Mobility*

  Seal canal with speculum, and gently apply positive (squeeze bulb) and negative (release bulb) pressure with pneumatic attachment.

  EXPECTED: Tympanic membrane moves in and out.

  UNEXPECTED: No movement of tympanic membrane.

Assess hearing

- *Questions asked during history*

  EXPECTED: Responds to questions appropriately.

  UNEXPECTED: Excessive requests for repetition. Speech with monotonous tone and erratic volume.

- *Whispered voice*
  Have patient mask hearing in one ear by inserting a finger in ear canal. Stand 1 to 2 feet from other ear and softly whisper three-letter and -number combinations (e.g., 3, T, 9 or 5, M, 2). Use a different letter number combination in other ear.

  EXPECTED: Patient repeats numbers and letters correctly more than 50% of time.
  UNEXPECTED: Patient unable to repeat whispered words.

- *Weber test*
  Place base of vibrating tuning fork on midline vertex of head. Repeat with one ear occluded.

  EXPECTED: Sound heard equally in both ears when ears are not occluded. Sound heard better in occluded ear.
  UNEXPECTED: See table on p. 81.

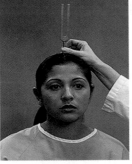

Weber test.

- *Rinne test*
  Place base of vibrating tuning fork against mastoid bone, note seconds until sound is no longer heard; then quickly move fork 1 to 2 cm ($^1/_2$ to 1 inch) from auditory canal and note seconds until sound is no longer heard. Repeat with other ear.

  EXPECTED: Measurement of air-conducted sound twice as long as measurement of bone- conducted sound.
  UNEXPECTED: See table on p. 81.

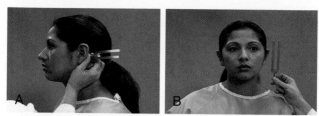

Rinne test. **A,** Tuning fork against mastoid bone. **B,** Tuning fork near ear.

Interpretation of Tuning Fork Tests

	Weber Test	Rinne Test
Expected findings	No lateralization, but will lateralize to ear occluded by patient	Air conduction heard longer than bone conduction by 2:1 ratio (Rinne positive)
Conductive hearing loss	Lateralization to deaf ear unless sensorineural loss	Bone conduction heard longer than air conduction in affected ear (Rinne negative)
Sensorineural hearing loss	Lateralization to better hearing ear unless conductive loss	Air conduction heard longer than bone conduction in affected ear, but <2:1 ratio

Nose and Sinuses

Inspect external nose

- *Shape/size*

  EXPECTED: Smooth. Columella directly midline, width is not greater than diameter of a naris.
  UNEXPECTED: Swelling or depression of nasal bridge. Transverse crease at junction of nose cartilage and bone.

- *Color*

  EXPECTED: Conforms to face color.

- *Nares*

  EXPECTED: Oval. Symmetrically positioned.
  UNEXPECTED: Asymmetry, narrowing, discharge, nasal flaring on inspiration.

Palpate ridge and soft tissues of nose
Place one finger on each side
of nasal arch and gently palpate from
nasal bridge to tip.

EXPECTED: Firm and stable
structures.
UNEXPECTED: Displacement of
bone and cartilage, tenderness, or
masses.

Evaluate patency of nares
Occlude one naris with finger
on side of nose, ask patient to breathe
through nose. Repeat
with other naris.

EXPECTED: Noiseless, easy
breathing.
UNEXPECTED: Noisy breathing;
occlusion.

Inspect nasal mucosa and nasal septum
Carefully tilt back the patient's
head and gently insert speculum without overdilating naris.

- *Color*

EXPECTED: Mucosa and turbinates
deep pink and glistening.
UNEXPECTED: Increased redness
of mucosa or localized redness and
swelling in vestibule. Turbinates
bluish gray or pale pink.

- *Shape*

EXPECTED: Septum close to
midline and fairly straight, thicker
anteriorly than posteriorly. Inferior
and middle turbinates visible.
UNEXPECTED: Asymmetry of
posterior nasal cavities, septal
deviation.

- *Condition*

EXPECTED: Possibly film of clear
discharge on septum. Possibly
hairs in vestibule. Turbinates firm
consistency.
UNEXPECTED: Discharge, bleeding,
crusting, masses, or lesions. Swollen, boggy turbinates. Perforated
septum. Polyps.

Sense of Smell
See Chapter 19.

Inspect frontal and maxillary sinus area

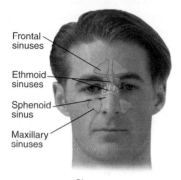

Frontal sinuses
Ethmoid sinuses
Sphenoid sinus
Maxillary sinuses

Sinuses.

UNEXPECTED: Swelling on face over sinus areas.

Palpate frontal and maxillary sinuses

Press thumbs up under bony brow on each side of nose.
Palpate with thumbs or index and middle fingers under zygomatic processes.

EXPECTED: Nontender on palpation.
UNEXPECTED: Tenderness or pain, swelling.

Mouth

Inspect and palpate lips with mouth closed

Have patient remove lipstick (if applicable).

* Symmetry

EXPECTED: Symmetric vertically and horizontally at rest and while moving.
UNEXPECTED: Asymmetric.

* Color

EXPECTED: Pink in persons with lighter skin, more bluish in persons with darker skin, distinct border between lips and facial skin.
UNEXPECTED: Pallor, circumoral pallor, bluish purple, or cherry red.

* Condition

EXPECTED: Smooth.
UNEXPECTED: Dry, cracked; deep fissures in mouth corners, swelling; lesions; plaques; vesicles; nodules; ulcerations; or round, oval, or irregular bluish gray macules.

Inspect teeth

- *Occlusion*

  Have patient clench teeth and smile with lips spread.

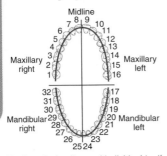

Teeth occlusion line and individual tooth numbers. *(From Miyasaki-Ching, 1997.)*

EXPECTED: Upper molars fit into the groove on lower molars. Premolars and canines interlock fully. Upper incisors slightly override lower incisors.
UNEXPECTED: Malocclusion. Protrusion of upper incisors (overbite). Protrusion of lower incisors. Problems with bite.

- *Color*

  EXPECTED: Ivory, stained yellow or brown.
  UNEXPECTED: Discolorations on crown may indicate caries.

- *Condition*

  EXPECTED: 32 teeth, firmly anchored.
  UNEXPECTED: Caries, and loose or missing teeth.

Inspect buccal mucosa

Have patient remove any dental appliances and then partially open mouth. Use tongue blade and bright light to assess.

- *Color*

  EXPECTED: Pinkish red, patchy pigmented mucosa in individuals with dark skin.
  UNEXPECTED: Deeply pigmented. Whitish or pinkish scars.

- *Condition*

  EXPECTED: Smooth and moist. Whitish yellow or whitish pink Stensen duct. Fordyce spots.
  UNEXPECTED: Adherent thickened white patch; white, round, or oval ulcerative lesions; red spot at opening of Stensen duct; stones or exudate from Stensen duct.

Inspect and palpate gingiva
Use gloves to palpate.

* *Color*

EXPECTED: Slightly stippled and pink, may be more hyperpigmented in individuals with dark skin.

* *Condition*

EXPECTED: Clearly defined, tight margin at each tooth. Gingival enlargement with pregnancy, puberty, certain medications.
UNEXPECTED: Inflammation, swelling, bleeding, or lesions under dentures or on gingiva; induration, thickening, masses, or tenderness. Enlarged crevices between teeth and gum margins. Pockets containing debris at tooth margins.

Inspect tongue
* *Size/symmetry*
Ask patient to extend tongue.

EXPECTED: Midline, no fasciculations.
UNEXPECTED: Atrophied, deviation to one side.

* *Color*
* *Dorsum surface*
Have patient extend tongue and hold extended.

EXPECTED: Dull red.
EXPECTED: Moist and glistening. Anterior: smooth yet roughened surface with papillae and small fissures. Posterior: smooth, slightly uneven or rugated surface with thinner mucosa than anterior. Possibly geographic.
UNEXPECTED: Smooth, red, slick; hairy; swollen; coated; ulcerated; fasciculations; or limitation of movement.

* *Ventral surface and floor of mouth*
  Have patient touch tip of tongue to palate behind upper incisors.

EXPECTED: Ventral surface pink and smooth with large veins between frenulum and fimbriated folds. Wharton ducts apparent on each side of frenulum.
UNEXPECTED: Difficulty touching hard palate. Swelling, varicosities, ranula (mucocele).

EARS, NOSE, AND THROAT

- *Lateral borders*
  Wrap tongue with gauze and pull to each side. Scrape white or red margins to remove food particles.

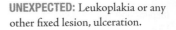
UNEXPECTED: Leukoplakia or any other fixed lesion, ulceration.

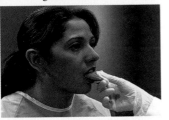

Inspecting lateral border of tongue.

Palpate tongue and floor of mouth

EXPECTED: Smooth and even texture.
UNEXPECTED: Lumps, nodules, induration, ulcerations, or thickened white patches.

Inspect palate and uvula
Have patient tilt head back.
- *Color and landmarks*

EXPECTED: Hard palate (whitish and dome-shaped with transverse rugae) contiguous with pinker soft palate. Uvula at midline. Bony protuberance of hard palate at midline (torus palatinus).
UNEXPECTED: Nodule on palate, not at midline.

- *Movement*
  Ask patient to say "ah" while observing soft palate. (Depress tongue if necessary.)

EXPECTED: Soft palate rises symmetrically, with uvula remaining in midline.
UNEXPECTED: Failure of soft palate to rise bilaterally. Uvula deviation. Bifid uvula.

Inspect oropharynx
Depress tongue with tongue blade.
- *Tonsils*
Inspect the tonsillar pillars and size of tonsils.

EXPECTED: Tonsils, if present, blend into pink color of pharynx. Possible crypts in tonsils where cellular debris and food particles collect.
UNEXPECTED: Tonsils projecting beyond limits of tonsillar pillars. Tonsils red, enlarged, covered with exudate.

- *Posterior wall of pharynx*

EXPECTED: Smooth, glistening, pink mucosa with some small, irregular spots of lymphatic tissue and small blood vessels.
UNEXPECTED: Red bulge adjacent to tonsil extending beyond midline. Yellowish mucoid film in pharynx.

Elicit gag reflex
Prepare patient and touch posterior wall of pharynx on each side.

EXPECTED: Bilateral response.
UNEXPECTED: Unequal response or no response.

AIDS TO DIFFERENTIAL DIAGNOSIS

Differentiating Between Otitis Externa, Acute Otitis Media, and Middle-Ear Effusion

Signs and Symptoms	Otitis Externa	Acute Otitis Media	Otitis Media with Effusion
Initial symptoms	Itching in ear canal	Abrupt onset, fever, irritability, feeling of blockage	Sticking or cracking sound on yawning or swallowing; no signs of acute infection
Pain	Intense with movement of pinna or chewing	Deep-seated earache that interferes with activity or sleep, pulling at ear	Discomfort; feeling of fullness
Discharge	Watery, then purulent and thick, mixed with pus and epithelial cells; musty, foul smelling	Only if tympanic membrane ruptures or through tympanostomy; tube; foul smelling	Uncommon
Hearing	Conductive loss caused by exudate and swelling of ear canal	Conductive loss as middle ear fills with pus	Conductive loss as middle ear fills with fluid

Differentiating Between Otitis Externa, Acute Otitis Media, and Middle-Ear Effusion—cont'd

Signs and Symptoms	Otitis Externa	Acute Otitis Media	Otitis Media with Effusion
Inspection	Canal is red, edematous; tympanic membrane is obscured	Tympanic membrane with distinct erythema, thickened or clouding, bulging; limited movement to positive and negative pressure, air–fluid level, and/or bubbles	Tympanic membrane is retracted or bulging, yellowish; impaired mobility; air–fluid level and/or bubbles

Subjective Data	Objective Data
Otitis Externa Swimming underwater, water retained in ear canal.	See differential diagnosis table on pp. 87-88.
Otitis Media with Effusion Upper respiratory infection, ear feels full, reduced hearing.	See differential diagnosis table on pp. 87-88.
Acute Otitis Media Recent upper respiratory infection, fever, ear pain or pressure, reduced hearing.	See differential diagnosis table on pp. 87-88.
Sinusitis Upper respiratory infection worsens after 5 days and persists for 10 days, headache, facial pain or pressure, tooth pain, nasal discharge or congestion, persistent cough.	Fever, tenderness of sinuses, swelling over orbit or sinus; purulent nasal discharge; dull or opaque transillumination.
Acute Pharyngitis, Tonsillitis Sore throat, referred pain to ears, dysphagia, fever, fetid breath, malaise.	Tonsils are red and swollen; crypts filled with purulent exudate; enlarged anterior cervical lymph nodes; palatal petechiae.

Peritonsillar Abscess

Difficulty swallowing, severe sore throat with pain radiating to ear, fever, malaise.

Drooling, unilateral red and swollen tonsil and adjacent soft palate; tonsil, may appear pushed forward or backward, possibly displacing uvula; muffled voice, fetid breath, trismus, enlarged cervical lymph nodes.

Retropharyngeal Abscess

Recent upper respiratory infection, pain in neck and jaw referred to ear, drooling, poor appetite.

Fever, restlessness, pain with lateral neck movement, lateral pharyngeal wall is distorted medially, trismus, respiratory distress, muffled voice.

Oral Cancer

Uses tobacco products, painless sore in mouth that does not heal.

Ulcerative lesion (red, white, pigmented) on lateral border of tongue, floor of mouth, or other mucosa. Firm nonmobile mass, tooth mobility when no periodontal disease present; cervical lymphadenopathy.

Periodontal Disease

Red, swollen gums that easily bleed, tender gums, loose teeth, teeth sensitive to temperature.

Plaque and tartar buildup on teeth, deep pockets between teeth and gum margins, loose or missing teeth, halitosis.

PEDIATRIC VARIATIONS

EXAMINATION

Technique	Findings

Ears

Inspect tympanic membrane
In infants, pull auricle downward and back to straighten canal.

EXPECTED: Tympanic membrane may be red from crying. If red from crying, it will be mobile.

Assess hearing
Evaluate response to auditory stimuli (tissue paper, whispered voice). Whisper words child recognizes like Big Bird, Donald Duck, and SpongeBob.

EXPECTED: For infants, see table on p. 90. Young children should turn toward sound consistently. Children repeat words whispered.

EARS, NOSE, AND THROAT

Sequences of Expected Hearing and Speech Response in Infants

Age	Response
Birth to 3 mo	Startles, wakes, or cries when hearing a loud sound; quiets to parent's voice; makes vowel sounds "oh" and "ah."
4-6 mo	Turns head toward interesting sound; moves eyes in direction of sound but may not always recognize location of sound; responds to parent's voice; enjoys sound-producing toys; starts babbling with many speech sounds.
7-12 mo	Responds to own name, telephone ringing, and person's voice, even if not loud; localizes sounds on all planes by turning eyes and head toward sound; babbles with short and long strings of sounds; begins to imitate speech sounds.

Modified from American Speech Language and Hearing Association: *How Does Your Child Hear and Talk*, 2012. Retrieved from http://www.asha.org/public/speech/development/01.htm.

Technique	Findings

Nose and Sinuses

Evaluate patency of nares

With infant's mouth closed or with infant sucking on bottle or pacifier, occlude one naris and then the other. Observe respiratory pattern.

EXPECTED: Breathes easily; obligatory nose breathing until 2-3 mo of age.

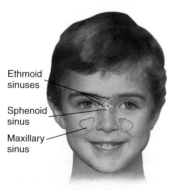

Ethmoid sinuses

Sphenoid sinus

Maxillary sinus

Pediatric sinuses.

Mouth

Inspect and palpate lips with mouth closed

EXPECTED: Drooling in infants age 6 wk to 6 mo, sucking calluses in newborns.
UNEXPECTED: Drooling persistent after age 6 mo not associated with teething.

Inspect teeth
Ask child to let you see his or her teeth.

EXPECTED: 0-20 teeth until age 6 years. Permanent teeth start erupting around age 6 years.
UNEXPECTED: Natal teeth.

Inspect buccal mucosa

EXPECTED: In infants, nonadherent white patches (milk).
UNEXPECTED: In infants, adherent white patches.

Inspect and palpate gingiva

EXPECTED: In infants up to 2 mo, pearl-like retention cysts.

Inspect and palpate hard palate

EXPECTED: Strong suck and Epstein pearls in young infants.
UNEXPECTED: No cleft of hard or soft palate.

AIDS TO DIFFERENTIAL DIAGNOSIS

Subjective Data	Objective Data
Cleft Lip and Palate	
Difficulty sucking, formula comes out of nose, failure to gain weight.	Unilateral or bilateral fissure or cleft in lip, hard palate, or soft palate that extends into the nasal cavity.

SAMPLE DOCUMENTATION

Subjective. A 55-year-old man has concerns about hearing loss for the past few months; it is particularly difficult to hear people talking. He has difficulty hearing on phone and when in conversations with multiple people talking. He hears "noise" in both ears when trying to go to sleep at night. There is no ear pain or discharge, no nasal discharge or sinus pain, no mouth lesions or masses, no recent dental problems, no sore throat, and no head trauma or exposure to ototoxic medications.

Objective. *Ears:* Auricles in alignment without masses, lesions, or tenderness. Canals totally obstructed by cerumen bilaterally. After irrigation, tympanic membranes are pearly gray, noninjected, intact, with bony landmarks and light reflex visualized bilaterally. No evidence of fluid or retraction. Conversational hearing appropriate. Able to hear whispered voice. Weber—lateralizes equally to both ears; Rinne—air conduction greater than bone conduction bilaterally (30 sec/15 sec).

Nose: No discharge or polyps, mucosa pink and moist, septum midline, patent bilaterally. No edema over frontal or maxillary sinuses. No sinus tenderness to palpation.

Mouth: Buccal mucosa pink and moist without lesions. Twenty-six teeth present in various states of repair. Lower second molars (18, 30) absent bilaterally. Gingiva pink and firm. Tongue midline with no tremors or fasciculation. Pharynx clear without erythema; tonsils 1+ without exudate. Uvula rises evenly and gag reflex is intact. No hoarseness.

CHAPTER 10

Chest and Lungs

EQUIPMENT

- Drape
- Skin-marking pencil
- Ruler and tape measure
- Stethoscope with bell and diaphragm

EXAMINATION

Have patient sit, disrobed to waist.

Technique	Findings

Chest and Lungs

Inspect front and back of chest
See thoracic landmarks.

- *Size/shape/symmetry*
- *Landmarks* — **EXPECTED:** Supernumerary nipples possible (can be clue to other congenital abnormalities, particularly in white individuals).

- *Compare anteroposterior diameter with transverse diameter* — **EXPECTED:** Ribs prominent, clavicles prominent superiorly, sternum usually flat and free of abundance of overlying tissue. Chest somewhat asymmetric. Anteroposterior diameter often half of transverse diameter.
  UNEXPECTED: Barrel chest, posterior or lateral deviation, pigeon chest, or funnel chest.

- *Assess nails, lips, nares* — **UNEXPECTED:** Clubbed fingernails (usually symmetric and painless; may indicate disease, may be hereditary), pursed lips, flared alae nasi.

- *Color*
  Assess skin, lips, and nails. — **UNEXPECTED:** Superficial venous patterns. Cyanosis or pallor of lips or nails.
- *Breath* — **UNEXPECTED:** Malodorous.

CHEST AND LUNGS

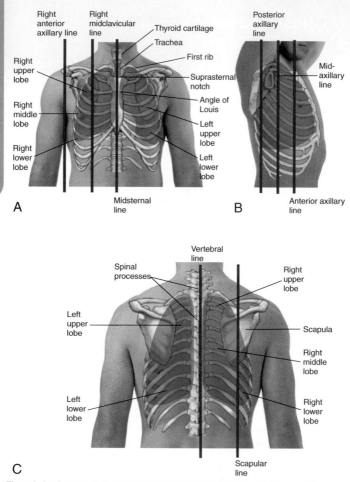

Thoracic landmarks. **A,** Anterior thorax. **B,** Right lateral thorax. **C,** Posterior thorax.

Evaluate respirations
• *Rhythm or pattern and rate*
See patterns of respiration in figure below.

EXPECTED: Breathing easy, regular, without distress. Pattern even. Rate 12-20 respirations/min. Ratio of respirations to heartbeats about 1:4.
UNEXPECTED: Dyspnea, orthopnea, paroxysmal nocturnal dyspnea, platypnea, tachypnea, hypopnea. Use of accessory muscles, retractions.

CHEST AND LUNGS

Normal	Regular and comfortable at a rate of 12-20 per minute	Air trapping	Increasing difficulty in getting breath out
Bradypnea	Slower than 12 breaths per minute	Cheyne-Stokes	Varying periods of increasing depth interspersed with apnea
Tachypnea	Faster than 20 breaths per minute	Kussmaul	Rapid, deep, labored
Hyperventilation (hyperpnea)	Faster than 20 breaths per minute, deep breathing	Biot	Irregularly interspersed periods of apnea in a disorganized sequence of breaths
Sighing	Frequently interspersed deeper breath	Ataxic	Significant disorganization with irregular and varying depths of respiration

Patterns of respiration. The horizontal axis indicates the relative rates of these patterns. The vertical swings of the lines indicate the relative depth of respiration.

• *Inspiration/expiration ratio*

UNEXPECTED: Air trapping, prolonged expiration.

Inspect chest movement with breathing
• *Symmetry*

EXPECTED: Chest expansion bilaterally symmetric.
UNEXPECTED: Asymmetry. Unilateral or bilateral bulging. Bulging on expiration.

Listen to respiration sounds audible without stethoscope

EXPECTED: Generally bronchovesicular.
UNEXPECTED: Crepitus, stridor, wheezes.

Palpate thoracic muscles and skeleton

- *Symmetry/condition*

EXPECTED: Bilateral symmetry. Some elasticity of rib cage, but sternum and xiphoid relatively inflexible and thoracic spine rigid.
UNEXPECTED: Pulsations, tenderness, bulges, depressions, unusual movement, unusual positions.

- *Thoracic expansion*
Stand behind patient. Place palms in light contact with posterolateral surfaces and thumbs along spinal processes at tenth rib, as shown in figure at right. Watch thumb divergence during quiet and deep breathing. Face patient; place thumbs along costal margin and xiphoid process with palms touching anterolateral chest. Watch thumb divergence during quiet and deep breathing.

EXPECTED: Symmetric expansion.

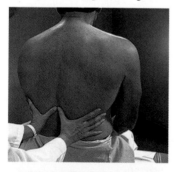

Palpating thoracic expansion. The thumbs are at the level of the tenth rib.

- *Sensations*

  UNEXPECTED: Asymmetric expansion.
  EXPECTED: Nontender sensations.
  UNEXPECTED: Crepitus or grating vibration.

- *Tactile fremitus*
  Ask patient to recite numbers or words while systematically palpating chest with palmar surfaces of fingers or ulnar aspect of clenched fist, using firm, light touch. Assess each area, front to back, side to side, lung apices. Compare sides.

  EXPECTED: Great variability; generally, fremitus is more intense with males (lower-pitched voice).
  UNEXPECTED: Decreased or absent fremitus; increased fremitus (coarser, rougher); or gentle, more tremulous fremitus. Variation between similar positions on right and left thorax.

Note position of trachea
Using index finger or thumbs, palpate gently from suprasternal notch along upper edges of each clavicle and in spaces above, to inner borders of sternocleidomastoid muscles.

EXPECTED: Spaces equal side to side. Trachea midline directly above suprasternal notch. Possible slight deviation to right.
UNEXPECTED: Significant deviation or tug. Pulsations.

Perform percussion on chest
Percuss as shown in figure below. Compare all areas bilaterally, following a sequence such as shown in figures on p. 98.
See table on p. 98 for common tones, intensity, pitch, duration, and quality.

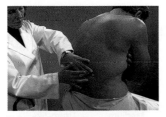

Method for percussion.

CHEST AND LUNGS

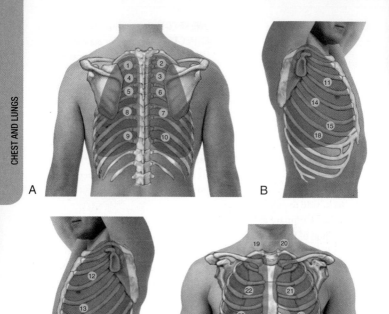

Suggested sequence for systematic percussion and auscultation of the thorax. **A,** Posterior thorax. **B,** Right lateral thorax. **C,** Left lateral thorax. **D,** Anterior thorax. The pleximeter finger or the stethoscope is moved in the numeric sequence suggested; however, other sequences are possible.

Percussion Tones Heard Over the Chest

Type of Tone	Intensity	Pitch	Duration	Quality
Resonant	Loud	Low	Long	Hollow
Flat	Soft	High	Short	Extremely dull
Dull	Medium	Medium-high	Medium	Thud-like
Tympanic	Loud	High	Medium	Drum-like
Hyperreso-nant*	Very loud	Very low	Longer	Booming

*Hyperresonance is unexpected in adults. It represents air trapping, which occurs in obstructive lung diseases.

Technique

- *Thorax*

  Have patient sit with head bent and arms folded in front while percussing posterior thorax, then with arms raised overhead while percussing lateral and anterior chest.

  Percuss at 4- to 5-cm intervals over intercostal spaces, moving superior to inferior, medial to lateral. The female breast may obscure findings. You or the patient may need to shift the breast, but pay careful attention to modesty.

- *Diaphragmatic excursion*

  Ask patient to breathe deeply and hold breath. Percuss along scapular line on one side until tone changes from resonant to dull. Mark skin.

  Allow patient to breathe normally, then repeat on other side. Have patient take several breaths, then exhale as much as possible and hold. On each side, percuss up from mark to change from dull to resonant.

  Tell patient to resume breathing comfortably. Measure excursion distance.

Findings

EXPECTED: Resonance over all areas of lungs, dull over heart and liver, spleen, areas of thorax.
UNEXPECTED: Hyperresonance, dullness, or flatness.

EXPECTED: 3-5 cm (higher on right than left).
UNEXPECTED: Limited descent.

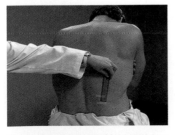

Measuring diaphragmatic excursion.
Excursion distance is usually 3 to 5 cm.

Auscultate chest with stethoscope diaphragm, apex to base

- *Intensity, pitch, duration, and quality of breath sounds*

  Have patient breathe slowly and deeply through mouth.

  Follow set auscultation sequence, holding stethoscope as shown in figure below.

  Ask patient to sit upright:
  - (1) with head bent and arms folded in front while auscultating posterior thorax.
  - (2) with arms raised overhead while auscultating lateral chest.
  - (3) with arms down and shoulders back while auscultating anterior chest.

  Listen during inspiration and expiration. Auscultate downward from apex to base at intervals of several centimeters, making side- to-side comparisons.

EXPECTED: See expected breath sounds in table on p. 101.

UNEXPECTED: Amphoric or cavernous breathing. Sounds difficult to hear or absent. Crackles, rhonchi, wheezes, or pleural friction rub, as described in box on pp. 101-102.

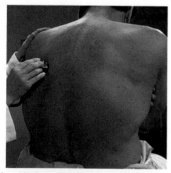

Auscultation with a stethoscope.

- *Vocal resonance*
  Ask patient to recite numbers or words.

EXPECTED: Muffled and indistinct sounds.
UNEXPECTED: Bronchophony, whispered pectoriloquy, or egophony.

Characteristics of Expected Breath Sounds

Sound	Characteristics	Findings
Vesicular	Heard over most of lung fields; low pitch; soft and short expirations; will be accentuated in a thin person or a child and diminished in overweight or very muscular patient.	
Bronchovesicular	Heard over main bronchus area and over upper right posterior lung field; medium pitch; expiration equals inspiration.	
Bronchotracheal (tubular)	Heard only over trachea; high pitch; loud and long expirations, often somewhat longer than inspiration.	

Adventitious Breath Sounds

Fine crackles: High-pitched, discrete, discontinuous crackling sounds heard during end of inspiration; not cleared by cough.

Medium crackles: Lower, more moist sound heard during mid-stage of inspiration; not cleared by cough.

Coarse crackles: Loud, bubbly noise heard during inspiration; not cleared by cough.

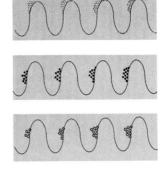

CHEST AND LUNGS

Rhonchi (sonorous wheeze):
Loud, low, coarse sounds, like
a snore, most often heard continuously during inspiration or
expiration; coughing may clear
sound (usually means mucus
accumulation in trachea or large
bronchi).

Wheeze (sibilant wheeze):
Musical noise sounding like a
squeak; most often heard continuously during inspiration or
expiration; usually louder during
expiration.

Pleural friction rub: Dry rubbing or
grating sound, usually caused by
inflammation of pleural surfaces;
heard during inspiration or expiration; loudest over lower lateral
anterior surface.

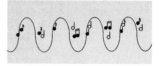

AIDS TO DIFFERENTIAL DIAGNOSIS

Subjective Data

Objective Data

Pleural Effusion

Cough with progressive dyspnea
is the typical presenting concern.
Pleuritic chest pain occurs with an
inflammatory effusion.

Findings on auscultation and percussion vary with the amount of fluid
present and with the position of
the patient. These include dullness
to percussion and tactile fremitus,
which are the most useful findings
for pleural effusion. When the fluid
is mobile it will gravitate to the most
dependent position. In the affected
areas, the breath sounds are muted
and the percussion note is often
hyperresonant in the area above the
perfusion.

Lung Cancer

Cough, wheezing, a variety of patterns of emphysema and atelectasis, pneumonitis, and hemoptysis. Peripheral tumors without airway obstruction may be asymptomatic.

Findings are based on the extent of the tumor and the patterns of its invasion and metastasis. With airway obstruction a postobstructive pneumonia can develop with consolidation. A malignant pleural effusion may develop with corresponding findings.

Pneumonia

Rapid onset (hours to days) of cough, pleuritic chest pain, and dyspnea. Sputum production is common with bacterial infection (see table on p. 104). Chills, fever, rigors, and nonspecific abdominal symptoms of nausea and vomiting may be present. Involvement of the right lower lobe can stimulate the tenth and eleventh thoracic nerves to cause right lower quadrant pain and simulate an abdominal process.

Febrile, tachypneic, and tachycardic. Crackles and rhonchi are common with diminished breath sounds. Egophony, bronchophony, and whisper pectoriloquy. Dullness to percussion occurs over the area of consolidation.

Asthma

Episodes of paroxysmal dyspnea and cough. Chest pain is common and, with it, a feeling of tightness. Episodes may last for minutes, hours, or days. May be asymptomatic between episodes.

Tachypnea with wheezing on expiration and inspiration. Expiration becomes more prolonged with labored breathing, fatigue, and anxious expression as airway resistance increases. Hypoxemia by pulse oximetry.

Chronic Bronchitis

Dyspnea may be present, although not severe. Cough and sputum production are impressive.

Wheezing and crackles. Hyperinflation with decreased breath sounds and a flattened diaphragm. Severe chronic bronchitis may result in right ventricular failure with dependent edema.

Emphysema

Dyspnea is common even at rest. Cough is infrequent without much production of sputum.

Chest may be barrel-shaped, and scattered crackles or wheezes may be heard. Overinflated lungs are hyperresonant on percussion. Inspiration is limited with a prolonged expiratory effort (i.e., >4 or 5 sec) to expel air.

Assessing Sputum

Cause	Possible Sputum Characteristics
Bacterial infection	Yellow, green, rust-colored (blood mixed with yellow sputum), clear, or transparent; purulent; blood streaked; mucoid, viscid
Viral infection	Mucoid, viscid; blood streaked (not common)
Chronic infectious disease	All of the above; particularly abundant in early morning; slight, intermittent blood streaking; occasionally large amounts of blood
Carcinoma	Slight, persistent blood streaking
Infarction	Blood clotted; large amounts of blood
Tuberculous cavity	Large amounts of blood

PEDIATRIC VARIATIONS

EXAMINATION

Technique	Findings

Chest and Lungs

Inspect front and back of chest

- *Compare anteroposterior diameter with transverse diameter*

EXPECTED: Infant's chest is expected to measure 2-3 cm less than head circumference.

Evaluate respirations
- *Rhythm or pattern and rate*

EXPECTED:

Age	Respirations per Minute
Newborn	30-80
1 yr	20-40
3 yr	20-30
6 yr	16-22
10 yr	16-20
17 yr	12-20

Perform direct or indirect percussion on chest

- *Thorax*

EXPECTED: Hyperresonance may be heard in children.

Auscultate chest with stethoscope diaphragm, apex to base

- *Intensity, pitch, duration, and quality of breath sounds*

EXPECTED: In infants and children, expect transmitted breath sounds throughout chest. Vesicular sound is accentuated in a child. Absent or diminished breath sounds are harder to detect.

SAMPLE DOCUMENTATION

SUBJECTIVE. A 45-year-old woman presents with cough and fever for 4 days. Cough is nonproductive, persistent, and worse when she lies down. She feels ill and short of breath. Her chest feels "heavy." Fever up to 38.3° C (101° F). Taking acetaminophen and nonprescription cough syrup without relief.

OBJECTIVE. Pulse 104 per minute, temperature 38.2° C, blood pressure 122/82, respirations 32 per minute and somewhat labored; no retractions or stridor. Minimal increase in anteroposterior diameter of chest, without kyphosis or other defect. Trachea in midline without tug. Thoracic expansion symmetric. No friction rubs or tenderness over ribs or other bony prominences. Over posterior left base, diminished tactile fremitus, dull percussion note, and on auscultation, crackles that do not clear with cough, diminished breath sounds. Remaining lung fields are clear and free of adventitious sounds, with resonant percussion tones. Diaphragmatic excursion 3 cm bilaterally.

CHAPTER 11

Heart

EQUIPMENT

- Tangential light source
- Skin-marking pencil
- Stethoscope with bell and diaphragm
- Centimeter ruler

EXAMINATION

Technique	Findings

Heart

Inspect precordium

Have patient supine, and keep light source tangential.

- *Apical impulse*

EXPECTED: Visible about midclavicular line in fifth left intercostal space. Sometimes visible only with patient sitting. **UNEXPECTED:** Visible in more than one intercostal space; exaggerated lifts or heaves.

Palpate precordium

- *Apical impulse*
  Have patient supine. With warm hands, gently feel precordium, using proximal halves of fingers held together or whole hand, as shown in figure on p. 107. Methodically move from apex to left sternal border, base, right sternal border, epigastrium, axillae.

EXPECTED: Gentle, brief impulse, palpable within radius of ≤1 cm, although often not felt. **UNEXPECTED:** Heave or lift, loss of thrust, displacement to right or left; thrill.

Technique	Findings

Locate sensation in terms of its intercostal space and relationship to midsternal, midclavicular, axillary lines.

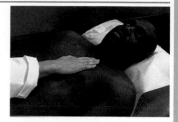

Percuss precordium (optional)

Begin by tapping at anterior axillary line, moving medially along intercostal spaces toward sternal borders until tone changes from resonance to dullness. Mark skin with marking pen.

EXPECTED: No change in tone before right sternal border; on left, loss of resonance generally close to point of maximal impulse at fifth intercostal space. Loss of resonance may outline left border of heart at second to fifth intercostal spaces.

Auscultate heart

Make certain patient is warm and relaxed. Isolate each sound and each pause in cycle, and then inch along with stethoscope. Systematically approach each of the five precordial areas, base to apex or apex to base, using each position shown in figures at right and below. Use diaphragm of stethoscope first, with firm pressure, then bell, with light pressure.

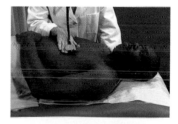

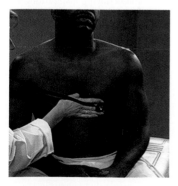

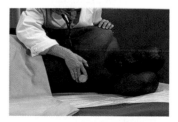

HEART

Technique	Findings

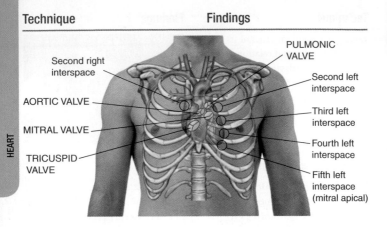

Second right interspace

AORTIC VALVE

MITRAL VALVE

TRICUSPID VALVE

PULMONIC VALVE

Second left interspace

Third left interspace

Fourth left interspace

Fifth left interspace (mitral apical)

- *Rate and rhythm*
  Assess overall rate and rhythm.

  EXPECTED: Rate 60-90 beats/min, regular rhythm.
  UNEXPECTED: Bradycardia, tachycardia, dysrhythmia.

- S_1
  Ask patient to breathe comfortably, then hold breath in expiration. Listen for S_1 (best heard toward apex) while palpating carotid pulse. Note intensity, variations, effect of respiration, splitting. Concentrate on systole, then diastole.

  EXPECTED: S_1 usually heard as one sound and coincides with rise of carotid pulse. See table on p. 109.
  UNEXPECTED: Extra sounds or murmurs.

- S_2
  Ask patient to breathe comfortably as you listen for S_2 (best heard in aortic and pulmonic areas) to become two components during inspiration. Ask patient to inhale and hold breath.

  EXPECTED: S_2 to become two components during inspiration. S_2 to become an apparent single sound as breath is exhaled. See table on p. 109.

- *Splitting*

  EXPECTED: S_2 splitting—greatest at peak of inspiration—varying from easily heard to nondetectable.

Technique	Findings
• S_3 and S_4 If needed, ask patient to raise a leg to increase venous return or to grip your hand vigorously and repeatedly to increase venous return.	**EXPECTED:** Both S_3 and S_4 quiet and difficult to hear. S_3 has rhythm of Ken-tuc-ky; S_4, Tenn-es-see. **UNEXPECTED:** Increased intensity (and ease of hearing) of either.
• Extra heart sounds	**UNEXPECTED:** Extra heart sounds—snaps, clicks, friction rubs, murmurs. See table on below.

Assess characteristics of murmurs

Timing and duration, pitch, intensity, pattern, quality, location, radiation, respiratory phase variations.

Heart Sounds According to Auscultatory Area

	Aortic	Pulmonic	Second Pulmonic	Mitral	Tricuspid
Pitch	$S_1 < S_2$	$S_1 < S_2$	$S_1 < S_2$	$S_1 > S_2$	$S_1 = S_2$
Loudness	$S_1 < S_2$	$S_1 < S_2$	$S_1 < S_2$*	$S_1 > S_2$†	$S_1 > S_2$
Duration	$S_1 < S_2$	$S_1 > S_2$	$S_1 < S_2$	$S_1 < S_2$	$S_1 = S_2$
S_2 split	>Inhale <Exhale	>Inhale <Exhale	>Inhale <Exhale	>Inhale† <Exhale	>Inhale <Exhale
A_2	Loudest	Loud	Decreased		
P_2	Decreased	Louder	Loudest		

*S_1 is relatively louder in second pulmonic area than in aortic area.
†S_1 may be louder in mitral area than in tricuspid area.
‡S_2 split may not be audible in mitral area if P_2 is inaudible.

Extra Heart Sounds

Sound	Detection	Description
Increased S_3	Bell at apex; patient left lateral recumbent	Early diastole, low pitch
Increased S_4	Bell at apex; patient supine or semilateral	Late diastole or early systole, low pitch
Gallops	Bell at apex; patient supine or left lateral recumbent	Presystole, intense, easily heard

Continued

HEART

Extra Heart Sounds—cont'd

Sound	Detection	Description
Mitral valve opening snap	Diaphragm medial to apex, may radiate to base; any position, second left intercostal	Early diastole briefly, before S_3; high pitch, sharp snap or click; not affected by respiration; easily confused with S_2
Ejection clicks	Diaphragm; patient sitting or supine	
Aortic valve	Diaphragm, right second intercostal space	Early systole, intense, high pitch; radiates, not affected by respirations
Pulmonary valve	Diaphragm; left second intercostal right space	Early systole, less intense than aortic click; intensifies on expiration, decreases on inspiration
Pericardial friction rub	Diaphragm, widely heard, sound clearest toward apex	May occupy all of systole and diastole; intense, grating, machine-like; may have three components and obliterate heart sounds; if only one or two components, may sound like murmur

AIDS TO DIFFERENTIAL DIAGNOSIS

Subjective Data	Objective Data
Left Ventricular Hypertrophy Initially asymptomatic, may cause shortness of breath or chest pain.	Vigorous, sustained lift palpable during ventricular systole, sometimes over broader area than usual (by ≥2 cm). Displacement of apical impulse can be well lateral of midclavicular line and downward.
Right Ventricular Hypertrophy Fatigue, shortness of breath, syncope may indicate more severe disease.	Lift along left sternal border in third and fourth left intercostal spaces accompanied by occasional systolic retraction at apex. Left ventricle displaced and turned posteriorly by enlarged right ventricle.

Subjective Data	Objective Data

Congestive Heart Failure
May be left or right sided:
Left sided is either systolic or diastolic.
Fatigue, orthopnea, shortness of breath, edema.

Congestion in pulmonary or systemic circulation. Can develop gradually or suddenly with acute pulmonary or systemic edema.

Cor Pulmonale
Tachypnea, fatigue, exertional dyspnea, cough hemoptysis.

Left parasternal systolic lift and loud S_2 in pulmonic region, evidence of pulmonary disease.

Myocardial Infarction
Deep substernal or visceral pain, often radiating to jaw, neck, left arm (although discomfort is sometimes mild); women may experience milder and different symptoms.

Dysrhythmias; S_4 often present. Heart sounds distant, with soft, systolic, blowing murmur; pulse possibly thready; varied blood pressure (although hypertension usual in early phases).

Myocarditis
Initially symptoms vague; fatigue, dyspnea, fever, palpitations. Symptoms may progress.

Cardiac enlargement, murmur, gallop rhythms, tachycardia, dysrhythmias, pulsus alternans.

Conduction Disturbances
Transient weakness, syncope, stroke-like episodes, palpitations.

Labile heart rates.

Atherosclerotic Heart Disease
May be asymptomatic or cause angina pectoris, shortness of breath, and palpitations.

May cause myocardial insufficiency, dysrhythmias, congestive heart failure.

Angina
Substernal pain or intense pressure radiating at times to neck, jaws, arms, particularly left arm, often accompanied by shortness of breath, fatigue, diaphoresis, faintness, syncope. Cessation of activity may relieve pain.

No pathognomonic examination findings, tachycardia, hypertension, diaphoresis, decreased S_1 intensity, S_4.

HEART

Chest Pain

Type of Chest Pain	Characteristics
Anginal	Substernal; provoked by effort, emotion, eating; relieved by rest and/or nitroglycerin
Pleural	Precipitated by breathing or coughing; usually described as sharp
Esophageal	Burning, substernal, occasional radiation to shoulder; nocturnal occurrence, usually when lying flat; relief with food, antacids, sometimes nitroglycerin
From a peptic ulcer	Almost always infradiaphragmatic and epigastric; nocturnal occurrence and daytime attacks; should not be relieved by food; unrelated to activity
Biliary	Usually under right scapula, prolonged in duration; will trigger angina more often than mimic it
From arthritis/bursitis	Usually of hours' long duration; local tenderness and/or pain with movement
Cervical	Associated with injury; provoked by activity, persists after activity; painful on palpation and/or movement
Musculoskeletal (chest)	Intensified or provoked by movement, particularly twisting or costochondral bending; long lasting; often associated with local tenderness
Psychoneurotic	Associated with or occurring after anxiety; poorly described, located in intramammary region

PEDIATRIC VARIATIONS

EXAMINATION

Technique	Findings
Assess characteristics of murmurs Timing and duration, intensity, pattern, quality, location, radiation, respiratory phase variations.	In children, it is necessary to distinguish innocent murmurs from organic murmurs caused by congenital defect or rheumatic fever.

AIDS TO DIFFERENTIAL DIAGNOSIS

Subjective Data	Objective Data

Chest Pain

Unlike in adults, chest pain in children and adolescents is seldom caused by a cardiac problem. It is very often difficult to find a cause, but trauma, exercise-induced asthma, and use of cocaine, even in a somewhat younger child, as in the adolescent and adult, should be among the considerations.

Examination is usually normal.

Congenital Defects

Tetralogy of Fallot

Dyspnea with feeding, poor growth, exercise intolerance, tetralogy spells.

Parasternal heave and precordial prominence, cyanosis, systolic ejection murmur heard over third intercostal space, sometimes radiating to left side of neck. Single S_2.

Ventricular septal defect

Tachypnea, symptoms of right-sided congestive heart failure, poor growth, recurrent respiratory infections.

Arterial pulse small, jugular venous pulse unaffected, regurgitation occurs through septal defect, resulting in holosystolic murmur that is frequently loud, coarse, high-pitched, best heard along left sternal border in third to fifth intercostal spaces. Distinct lift often discernible along left sternal border and apical area. Does not radiate to neck.

Subjective Data	Objective Data
Patent ductus arteriosus	
Asymptomatic if small; larger patent ductus arteriosi cause dyspnea on exertion.	Neck vessels dilate and pulsate, and pulse pressure wide. Harsh, loud, continuous murmur with machine-like quality, heard at first to third intercostal spaces and lower sternal border. Murmur usually unaltered by postural change.
Atrial septal defect	
Often asymptomatic, congestive heart failure in adults.	Systolic ejection murmur, best heard over pulmonic area that is diamond-shaped, often loud, high in pitch, and harsh. May be accompanied by brief, rumbling, early diastolic murmur. Does not usually radiate beyond precordium. Systolic thrill may be felt over area of murmur along with palpable parasternal thrust. S_2 may be split fairly widely. Particularly significant with palpable thrust and occasional radiation through to back.

SAMPLE DOCUMENTATION

Heart.   No visible pulsations over precordium. Point of maximal impulse palpable at the fifth intercostals in the midclavicular line, 1 cm in diameter. No lifts, heaves, or thrills felt on palpation. S_1 is crisp. Split S_2 increases with inspiration. No audible S_3, S_4, murmur, click, or rub.

CHAPTER 12

Blood Vessels

EQUIPMENT

- Tangential light source
- Stethoscope with bell and diaphragm
- Sphygmomanometer
- Centimeter ruler

EXAMINATION

Technique	Findings

Peripheral Arteries

Palpate arterial pulses in neck and extremities

Palpate carotid, brachial, radial, femoral, popliteal, dorsalis pedis, and posterior tibial arteries, using distal pads of second and third fingers, as shown in figures below and on p. 117.

- *Characteristics*
  Compare characteristics bilaterally, as well as between upper and lower extremities.

EXPECTED: Femoral pulse as strong as or stronger than radial pulse.
UNEXPECTED: Femoral pulse weaker than radial pulse or absent. Alternating pulse (pulsus alternans), pulsus bisferiens, bigeminal pulse (pulsus bigeminus), bounding pulse, labile pulse, paradoxical pulse (pulsus paradoxus), pulsus differens, tachycardia, trigeminal pulse (pulsus trigeminus), or water-hammer pulse (Corrigan pulse).

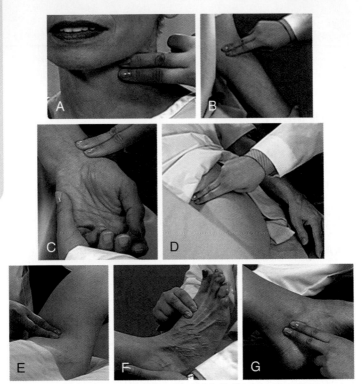

Palpation of arterial pulses. **A,** Carotid. **B,** Brachial. **C,** Radial. **D,** Femoral. **E,** Popliteal. **F,** Dorsalis pedis. **G,** Posterior tibial.

Technique	Findings
• *Rate*	**EXPECTED:** 60-90 beats/min. **UNEXPECTED:** Rate different from that observed during cardiac examination.
• *Rhythm*	**EXPECTED:** Regular. **UNEXPECTED:** Irregular, either in a pattern or patternless.
• *Contour*	**EXPECTED:** Smooth, rounded, or dome-shaped.

PULSE

POSSIBLE CAUSE

Alternating pulse (pulsus alternans)

Left ventricular failure
(More significant if
pulse slow)

A Pulsus alternans is characterized by alternation of a pulsation of small amplitude with the pulsation of large amplitude while the rhythm is regular.

Pulsus bisferiens

Aortic stenosis combined
with aortic insufficiency

B Pulsus bisferiens is best detected by palpation of the carotid artery. This pulsation is characterized by two main peaks. The first is termed percussion wave and the second, tidal wave. Although the mechanism is not clear, the first peak is believed to be the pulse pressure and the second, reverberation from the periphery.

Bigeminal pulse

Disorder of rhythm

C Bigeminal pulsations result from a normal pulsation followed by a premature contraction. The amplitude of the pulsation of the premature contraction is less than that of the normal pulsation.

Large, bounding pulse

Exercise
Anxiety
Fever
Hyperthyroidism
Aortic rigidity or
atherosclerosis

D The large, bounding (also called hyperkinetic or strong) pulse is readily palpable. It does not "fade out" and is not easily obliterated by the examining fingers. This pulse is recorded as 3+.

Paradoxic pulse (pulsus paradoxus)

Inspiration   Expiration   Inspiration

Premature cardiac contraction
Tracheobronchial obstruction
Bronchial asthma
Emphysema
Pericardial effusion
Constrictive pericarditis

E Pulsus paradoxus is characterized by an exaggerated decrease (>10 mm Hg) in the amplitude of pulsation during inspiration and increased amplitude during expiration. (See text for measurement with sphygmomanometer.)

Water-hammer pulse (Corrigan pulse)

Patent ductus arteriosus
Aortic regurgitation

F The water-hammer pulse (also known as collapsing) has a greater amplitude than expected, a rapid rise to a narrow summit, and a sudden descent.

A-F, Pulse abnormalities. *(Modified from Barkauskas et al, 2002.)*

Technique	Findings
• *Amplitude*	**UNEXPECTED:** Bounding, full, diminished, or absent. Describe on scale of 0-4: 0 = Absent, not palpable 1 = Diminished 2 = Expected 3 = Full, increased 4 = Bounding

Technique	Findings

Auscultate carotid and subclavian arteries; abdominal aorta; and renal, iliac, and femoral arteries for bruits

When auscultating the carotid vessels, you may at times need to ask patient to hold breath for a few heartbeats. Auscultate with bell of stethoscope.

UNEXPECTED: Transmitted murmurs, bruits.

Assess for arterial occlusion and insufficiency

- *Site*

  Assess for pain distal to possible occlusion.

UNEXPECTED: Dull ache accompanied by fatigue and often cramping; possible constant or excruciating pain. Weak, thready, or absent pulses; systolic bruits over arteries; loss of body warmth; localized pallor or cyanosis; delay in venous filling; or thin, atrophied skin, muscle atrophy, and loss of hair.

- *Degree of occlusion*

  Ask patient to lie supine.

  Elevate extremity, note degree of blanching, then ask patient to sit on edge of table or bed to lower extremity. Note time for maximal return of color when extremity is lowered.

EXPECTED: Slight pallor on elevation and return to full color as soon as leg becomes dependent.

UNEXPECTED: Delay of >2 sec.

Measure blood pressure

Measure in both arms at least once. Patient's arm should be slightly flexed and comfortably supported on table, pillow, or your hand.

EXPECTED: <120 mm Hg systolic and <80 mm Hg diastolic, with pulse pressure of 30-40 mm Hg (sometimes to 50 mm Hg). Reading between arms may vary by as much as 10 mm Hg. Prehypertension is now defined as a blood pressure between 120 and 139 mm Hg systolic or 80 and 89 mm Hg diastolic.

UNEXPECTED: Hypertension (see Chapter 2).

Technique	Findings

Peripheral Veins

Assess jugular venous pressure

Ask patient to recline at 45-degree angle. With tangential light, observe the jugular vein. As shown in figure below, use a centimeter ruler to measure vertical distance between midaxillary line and highest level of jugular vein distention.

EXPECTED: Pressure ≤9 cm H_2O, bilaterally symmetric.
UNEXPECTED: Abnormal elevation, distention or distention on one side.

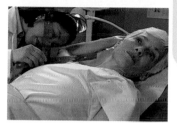

Assess for venous obstruction and insufficiency

Inspect extremities, with patient both standing and supine.

- *Affected area*

UNEXPECTED: Constant pain with swelling and tenderness over muscles, engorgement of superficial veins, cyanosis.

- *Thrombosis*
  Flex patient's knee slightly with one hand, and with other, dorsiflex foot to test for Homan sign.

UNEXPECTED: Redness, thickening, tenderness along superficial vein. Calf pain with test for Homan sign.

- *Edema*
  Press index finger over bony prominence of tibia or medial malleolus for several seconds.

UNEXPECTED: Orthostatic (pitting) edema; thickening and ulceration of skin possible.

Grade edema from 1+ to 4+ as follows:

    1+ = Slight pitting, no visible distortion, disappears rapidly

    2+ = Deeper than 1+ and disappears in 10-15 sec

    3+ = Noticeably deep and may last >1 min, with dependent extremity full and swollen

    4+ = Very deep and lasts 2-5 min, with grossly distorted dependent extremity

BLOOD VESSELS

Technique	Findings
• *Varicose veins* If suspected, have patient stand on toes 10 times in succession.	**EXPECTED:** Pressure from toe standing disappears in seconds. **UNEXPECTED:** Veins dilated and swollen; often tortuous when extremities are dependent and pressure does not quickly disappear.
• *If varicose veins are present, assess venous incompetence with Trendelenburg test:* Ask patient to lie supine, lift leg above heart level until veins empty, then quickly lower leg.	**UNEXPECTED:** Rapid filling of veins.
• *Evaluate patency of deep veins with Perthes test:* Ask patient to lie supine. Elevate extremity, and occlude subcutaneous veins with tourniquet just above knee. Then ask patient to walk.	**UNEXPECTED:** Superficial veins fail to empty.
• *Evaluate direction of blood flow and presence of compensatory circulation:* Put affected limb in dependent position, then empty or strip vein. Release pressure of one finger nearest heart to assess blood flow; if necessary, repeat and release pressure of other finger.	**UNEXPECTED:** Stripped vessel fills before pressure is released by distal finger, or blood refills entire vein when pressure is released by proximal finger.

AIDS TO DIFFERENTIAL DIAGNOSIS

Objective Data	Subjective Data
Arterial Aneurysm Generally asymptomatic until they dissect or compress an adjacent structure. With dissection, the patient may describe a severe ripping pain.	Pulsatile swelling along the course of an artery. Occurs most commonly in the aorta, although renal, femoral, and popliteal arteries are also common sites. A thrill or bruit may be evident over the aneurysm.

Objective Data	Subjective Data
Venous Thrombosis Tenderness along the iliac vessels or the femoral canal, in the popliteal space, or over the deep calf veins. Deep vein thrombosis in the femoral and pelvic circulations may be asymptomatic. Pulmonary embolism may occur without warning.	Swelling may be distinguished only by measuring and comparing the circumference of the upper and lower legs bilaterally. There may be minimal ankle edema, low-grade fever, and tachycardia. Homan sign can be helpful but is not absolutely reliable in suggesting deep vein thrombosis.
Raynaud Phenomenon Involved areas will feel cold and achy, which improves on rewarming. In secondary Raynaud phenomenon, there can be intense pain and digital ischemia with necrosis at the tips.	With primary Raynaud phenomenon, there is triphasic demarcated skin pallor (white), cyanosis (blue), and reperfusion (red) within the extremities. The vasospasm may last from minutes to less than an hour. In secondary Raynaud phenomenon, ulcers may appear on the tips of the digits, and eventually the skin over the digits can appear smooth, shiny, and tight from loss of subcutaneous tissue.

BLOOD VESSELS

PEDIATRIC VARIATIONS

EXAMINATION

Technique	Findings
Palpate arterial pulses in distal extremities (see Chapter 2)	
Auscultate arteries for bruits	
	EXPECTED: In children, it is not unusual to hear a venous hum over internal jugular veins. There is usually no pathologic significance.
Measure blood pressure (see Chapter 2)	

BLOOD VESSELS

AIDS TO DIFFERENTIAL DIAGNOSIS	
Subjective Data	Objective Data

Coarctation of the Aorta

Most patients are asymptomatic unless severe hypertension or vascular insufficiency develops. In those settings, patients may experience symptoms of heart failure or vascular insufficiency of an involved upper extremity with activity.

Differences in systolic blood pressure readings when the radial and femoral pulses are palpated simultaneously.

SAMPLE DOCUMENTATION

Vessels. Neck veins not distended. Both A and V waves are visualized. Jugular venous pressure (JVP) is 4 cm water at 45 degrees. Arterial pulses equal and symmetric, testing on a scale of 1-4.

	C	B	R	F	P	PT	DP
L	2 +	2 +	2 +	2 +	2 +	2 +	2 +
R	2 +	2 +	2 +	2 +	2 +	2 +	2 +

Vessels soft. No bruits are audible.

Extremities. No edema, skin, or nail changes. Superficial varicosities noted in both lower extremities. No areas of tenderness to palpation.

CHAPTER 13

Breasts and Axillae

EQUIPMENT

- Ruler (if mass detected)
- Flashlight with transilluminator (if mass detected)
- Glass slide and cytologic fixative (if nipple discharge is present)
- Small pillow or folded towel

EXAMINATION

Describe any breast mass or lump that you encounter using the following characteristics:

- Location: clock positions and distance from nipple
- Size (in centimeters): length, width, thickness
- Shape: round, discoid, lobular, stellate, regular or irregular
- Consistency: firm, soft, hard
- Tenderness
- Mobility: movable (in what directions) or fixed to overlying skin or sub adjacent fascia
- Borders: discrete or poorly defined
- Retraction: presence or absence of dimpling; altered contour

All new solitary or dominant masses must be investigated with further diagnostic testing.

Technique	Findings

Female Patients

With patient seated and arms hanging loosely, inspect both breasts

Inspect all quadrants and tail of Spence. If necessary, lift breasts with fingertips to expose lower and lateral aspects.

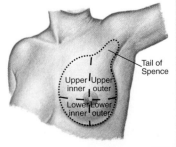

Tail of Spence

Upper inner | Upper outer

Lower inner | Lower outer

Technique	Findings
• Size/shape/symmetry	**EXPECTED:** Convex, pendulous, or conical. Frequently asymmetric in size.
• Texture/contour	**EXPECTED:** Smooth and uninterrupted.
	UNEXPECTED: Dimpling or peau d'orange appearance. Changes or asymmetric appearance.
• Skin color	**EXPECTED:** Consistent color
	UNEXPECTED: Areas of discoloration, erythema, or asymmetric appearance.
• Venous patterns	**EXPECTED:** Bilateral venous networks, although usually pronounced only in pregnant women.
	UNEXPECTED: Unilateral network.
• Markings	**EXPECTED:** Long-standing nevi. Supernumerary nipples possible (but could be a clue to other congenital abnormalities).
	UNEXPECTED: Changing or tender nevi. Lesions.
Inspect areolae and nipples	
• Size/shape/symmetry	**EXPECTED:** Areolae round or oval, bilaterally equal or nearly equal. Nipples bilaterally equal or nearly equal in size and usually everted, although one or both sometimes inverted.
	UNEXPECTED: Recent unilateral nipple inversion or retraction.
• Color	**EXPECTED:** Areolae and nipples pink to brown.
	UNEXPECTED: Nonhomogeneous in color.
• Texture/contour	**EXPECTED:** Areolae smooth, except for Montgomery tubercles. Nipples smooth or wrinkled.

Technique	Findings

UNEXPECTED: Areolae with suppurative or tender Montgomery tubercles or with peau d'orange appearance. Nipples crusting, cracking, or with discharge.

With patient in the following positions, reinspect both breasts

- *Arms extended over head or flexed behind the neck*

EXPECTED: All positions breasts bilaterally symmetric with even contour.

- *Hands pressed on hips with shoulders rolled forward or pushed together in front*

UNEXPECTED: Dimpling, retraction, deviation, or fixation of breasts.

- *Seated and leaning over*
- *Recumbent*

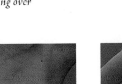

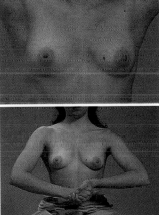

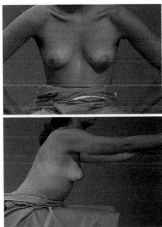

Technique	Findings

With patient seated and arms hanging loosely, palpate breasts

Chest wall sweep. Place the palm of your right hand at the patient's right clavicle at the sternum. Sweep downward from the clavicle to the nipple, feeling for superficial lumps. Repeat the sweep until you have covered the entire right chest wall. Repeat the procedure using your left hand for the left chest wall.

EXPECTED: Tissue smooth, free of lumps.
UNEXPECTED: Lumps or nodules. Reassess with additional palpation and characterize any masses by location, size, shape, consistency, tenderness, mobility, delineation of borders, retraction. Use transillumination to assess presence of fluid in masses.

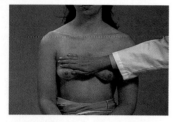

Bimanual digital palpation. Place one hand, palmar surface facing up, under the patient's right breast. Position your hand so that it acts as a flat surface against which to compress the breast tissue. Walk the fingers of the other hand across the breast tissue, feeling for lumps as you compress the tissue between your fingers and your flat hand. Repeat the procedure for the other breast.

EXPECTED: Tissue generally firm, nontender, free of lumps. During menstrual cycle, cyclic pattern of breast enlargement, increased nodularity, tenderness.
UNEXPECTED: Lumps or nodules. Reassess with additional palpation and characterize any masses by location, size, shape, consistency, tenderness, mobility, delineation of borders, retraction. Use transillumination to assess presence of fluid in masses.

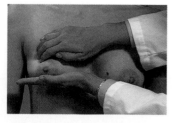

Technique	Findings

With patient seated, palpate for lymph nodes

Axillary: Support patient's forearm with your contralateral arm and bring palm of examining hand flat into axilla. With palmar surface of fingers, reach deep into hollow, pushing firmly upward, then bring fingers down, rotating your fingers and gently rolling soft tissue against chest wall and axilla. Explore apex, medial, lateral aspects along rib cage; lateral aspects along upper surface of arm; and anterior and posterior walls of axilla. Repeat mirror image of this maneuver for the other axilla.

EXPECTED: Nodes not palpable.
UNEXPECTED: Nodes, especially in supraclavicular area. Describe nodes by location, size, shape, consistency, tenderness, fixation, delineation of borders.

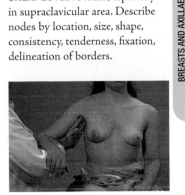

Supraclavicular area: Hook fingers over clavicle and rotate over supraclavicular fossa while patient turns head toward same side and raises shoulder.

Infraclavicular area: Palpate along the clavicle using a rotary motion with your fingers.

With patient supine, continue palpation of breast tissue

Have patient put one hand behind head. Place a towel under shoulder of same side. Compress breast tissue between fingers and chest wall, using rotary motion of fingers. Using finger pads, systematically palpate each breast in all four quadrants, including tail of Spence and over areolae. Push gently but firmly toward chest while rotating fingers clockwise or counterclockwise, following a vertical strip, concentric circle, or wedge pattern.

At each point, press inward, using three depths of palpation: light, medium, and deep.

EXPECTED: Tissue generally dense, firm, elastic but sometimes lobular. May be fine and granular in older women. Inframammary ridge may be felt along lower edge of breast. During menstrual cycle, cyclic pattern of breast enlargement, increased nodularity, tenderness.
UNEXPECTED: Lumps or nodules. Characterize any masses by location, size, shape, consistency, tenderness, mobility, delineation of borders, retraction. Use transillumination to assess presence of fluid in masses.

BREASTS AND AXILLAE

Technique	Findings
Return to the nipple and with two fingers gently depress the tissue inward into the well behind the areola. Repeat palpation maneuvers for other breast.	**EXPECTED:** Fingers and tissue move easily inward. **UNEXPECTED:** Lump, mass; absence of well behind areola.

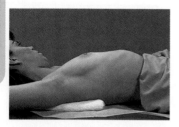 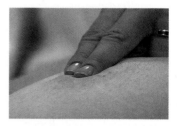

Male Patients

Inspect both breasts

- *Size/shape/symmetry*

EXPECTED: Even with chest wall. Sometimes convex (especially in overweight men).

- *Surface characteristics*

UNEXPECTED: Enlarged breasts.

Inspect areolae and nipples

- *Size/shape/symmetry*

EXPECTED: Areolae round or oval, bilaterally equal or nearly equal. Nipples bilaterally equal or nearly equal in size and usually everted, although one or both sometimes inverted.

UNEXPECTED: Recent unilateral nipple inversion or retraction.

- *Color*

EXPECTED: Areolae and nipples pink to brown.

UNEXPECTED: Nonhomogeneous in color.

- *Texture/contour*

EXPECTED: Areolae smooth, except for Montgomery tubercles. Nipples smooth or wrinkled.

UNEXPECTED: Areolae with suppurative or tender Montgomery tubercles or with peau d'orange appearance. Nipples crusting, cracking, or with discharge.

Technique	Findings
Palpate breasts and over areolae	
• *Palpate briefly, following palpation steps for female patients.*	**EXPECTED:** Thin layer of fatty tissue overlying muscle. Thick layer in obese men may give appearance of breast enlargement. Firm disk of glandular tissue sometimes evident. **UNEXPECTED:** Lumps or nodules
With patient seated and arms flexed at elbows, palpate for lymph nodes	
• *Palpate as described for female patients.*	**UNEXPECTED:** Nodes, especially in supraclavicular area. Describe nodes by location, size, shape, consistency, tenderness, fixation, delineation of borders.

AIDS TO DIFFERENTIAL DIAGNOSIS

Subjective Data	Objective Data
Fibrocystic Changes Tender and painful breasts and/or palpable lumps that fluctuate with menses; usually worse premenstrually	Round, soft to firm, tense, mobile masses with well-delineated borders; usually tender; usually bilateral; multiple or single.
Fibroadenoma Painless lumps that do not fluctuate with the menstrual cycle; may be asymptomatic with discovery on clinical breast examination or mammogram.	Round or discoid, firm, rubbery, mobile masses with well-delineated borders; usually nontender, usually bilateral, single; may be multiple; biopsy often performed to rule out carcinoma.
Malignant Breast Tumors Painless lump, change in size, shape or contour of breast, axilla may be tender if lymph nodes involved; may be asymptomatic with discovery on clinical breast examination or mammogram.	Palpable mass that is usually single, unilateral, irregular, or stellate in shape; poorly delineated borders; fixed, hard, stone-like, and non-tender; breast may have dimpling, retraction, prominent vasculature; skin may have peau d'orange or thickened appearance; nipple may be inverted or deviate in position.

BREASTS AND AXILLAE

Subjective Data	Objective Data

Intractal Papillomas and Papillomatosis

Spontaneous nipple discharge, usually unilateral; usually serous or bloody.

Single-duct unilateral nipple discharge provoked on physical examination.

Gynecomastia

Breast enlargement in male individuals.

Smooth, firm, mobile, tender disk of breast tissue behind areola, unilaterally or bilaterally.

Mastitis

Sudden onset of swelling, tenderness, redness, and heat in the breast; usually chills, fever.

Tender, hard breast mass, with an area of fluctuation, erythema, and heat; may have discharge of pus (suppuration).

PEDIATRIC VARIATIONS

EXAMINATION

Technique	Findings

Palpate and compress nipples

EXPECTED: Breast enlargement is not unusual in newborns. "Witch's milk" may be expressed.

Assess stage of pubertal development

In female patients, assess the stage of breast development.

EXPECTED: The duration and tempo of each stage and sequence are quite variable between individuals. Tanner stages of breast development are shown on p. 131.

M₁—Tanner 1 (preadolescent). Only the nipple is raised above the level of the breast, as in the child.

M₂—Tanner 2. Budding stage; bud-shaped elevation of the areola; areola increased in diameter and surrounding area slightly elevated.

M₃—Tanner 3. Breast and areola enlarged. No contour separation.

M₄—Tanner 4. Increasing fat deposits. The areola forms a secondary elevation above that of the breast. This secondary mound occurs in approximately half of all girls and in some cases persists in adulthood.

M₅—Tanner 5 (adult stage). The areola is (usually) part of general breast contour and is strongly pigmented. Nipple projects.

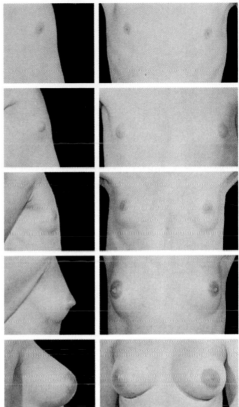

Five stages of breast development in females. *(Growth diagrams 1965 Netherlands: second national survey on 0-24-year-olds, by J. C. Van Wieringen, F. Wafelbakker, H. P. Verbrugge, J. H. DeHaas. Groningen: Noordhoff Uitgevers BV, The Netherlands.)*

AIDS TO DIFFERENTIAL DIAGNOSIS

Subjective Data	Objective Data
Premature thelarche	
Breast enlargement before onset of puberty	Degree of enlargement varies from very slight to fully developed breasts. Usually bilateral. Other signs of sexual maturation may be absent.

BREASTS AND AXILLAE

SAMPLE DOCUMENTATION

Subjective. A 42-year-old woman noticed a "knot" in her right lower breast last week. Denies nipple discharge or skin changes. Reports normal mammogram last year. Has never had a breast lump before. Currently on last day of menses. Has breast tenderness just before menses but denies breast pain today. No family history of breast cancer.

Objective. Breasts moderate size, conical shape, left slightly larger than right. No skin lesions, contour smooth without dimpling or retraction; venous pattern symmetric. Nipples symmetric, without spontaneous discharge, depress into the wells easily. Montgomery tubercles bilaterally. Breasts diffusely nodular, particularly in upper outer quadrants. In right breast there is a 3 × 2-cm soft, mobile, nontender mass with discrete, well-defined borders at the 4-o'clock position 6 cm from the nipple. No supraclavicular, infraclavicular, or axillary lymphadenopathy.

CHAPTER 14

Abdomen

EQUIPMENT

- Stethoscope
- Centimeter ruler and measuring tape
- Marking pen

EXAMINATION

Have patient in the supine position to start the examination. Approach the patient from the right side.

Technique	Findings
Inspect abdomen • *Skin color/characteristics*	**EXPECTED:** Usual color variations, such as paleness or tanning lines. Fine venous network (venous return toward head above umbilicus, toward feet below umbilicus). **UNEXPECTED:** Generalized color changes, such as jaundice or cyanosis. Glistening, taut appearance. Bluish periumbilical discoloration, bruises, other localized discoloration. Striae, lesions or nodules, a pearl-like enlarged umbilical node, scars.
• *Contour/symmetry* Begin seated to patient's right to enhance shadows and contouring. Inspect while patient breathes comfortably and while patient holds a deep breath. Assess symmetry, first seated at patient's side, then standing behind patient's head.	**EXPECTED:** Flat, rounded, or scaphoid. Contralateral areas symmetric. Maximum height of convexity at umbilicus. Abdomen remains smooth and symmetric while patient holds breath.

ABDOMEN

Technique	Findings
	UNEXPECTED: Umbilicus displaced upward, downward, or laterally or is inflamed, swollen, or bulging. Any distention (symmetric or asymmetric), bulges, or masses while breathing comfortably or holding breath.
• *Surface motion*	**EXPECTED:** Smooth, even motion with respiration. Female patients mostly costal movement; male patients mostly abdominal. Pulsations often visible in upper midline in thin adults.
	UNEXPECTED: Limited motion with respiration in male adults. Rippling movement (peristalsis) or marked pulsations.

Anatomic Correlates of the Four Quadrants of the Abdomen

Right Upper Quadrant	Left Upper Quadrant
Liver and gallbladder	Left lobe of liver
Pylorus	Spleen
Duodenum	Stomach
Head of pancreas	Body of pancreas
Right adrenal gland	Left adrenal gland
Portion of right kidney	Portion of left kidney
Hepatic flexure of colon	Splenic flexure of colon
Portions of ascending and transverse colon	Portions of transverse and descending colon

Right Lower Quadrant	Left Lower Quadrant
Lower pole of right kidney	Lower pole of left kidney
Cecum and appendix	Sigmoid colon
Portion of ascending colon	Portion of descending colon
Bladder (if distended)	Bladder (if distended)
Ovary and salpinx	Ovary and salpinx
Uterus (if enlarged)	Uterus (if enlarged)
Right spermatic cord	Left spermatic cord
Right ureter	Left ureter

Inspect abdominal muscles as patient raises head

EXPECTED: No masses or protrusions.

UNEXPECTED: Masses, protrusion of the umbilicus and other hernia signs, or separation of rectus abdominis.

Auscultate with stethoscope diaphragm

- *Frequency and character of bowel sounds*
  Warm stethoscope diaphragm and hold with light pressure.
  May auscultate at a single site because bowel sounds generalize, but auscultate in all quadrants if you have reason to be concerned.

EXPECTED: 5-35 irregular clicks and gurgles per minute. Borborygmi, or increased sounds, may be because of hunger.

UNEXPECTED: Increased sounds unrelated to hunger and high-pitched tinkling sounds may be caused by early intestinal obstruction; decreased or absent sounds after 5 min of listening may be associated with abdominal pain and rigidity.

- *Liver and spleen*

EXPECTED: Silent.

UNEXPECTED: Friction rubs (high-pitched grating sound in association with respiration).

Auscultate with stethoscope bell

- *Vascular sounds*
  Listen with stethoscope bell in epigastric region, over aorta, and over renal, iliac, and femoral arteries.

EXPECTED: No bruits (harsh or musical sound indicating blood flow turbulence), venous hum (soft, low-pitched, and continuous sound), or friction rubs.

UNEXPECTED: Bruits in aortic, renal, iliac, or femoral arteries.

- *Epigastric region and around umbilicus*

EXPECTED: No venous hum.

UNEXPECTED: Venous hum.

ABDOMEN

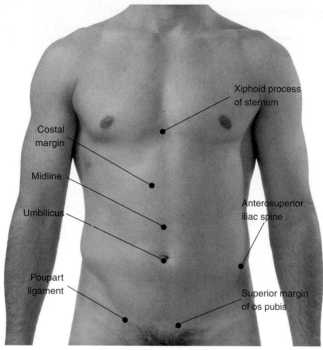

Xiphoid process
of sternum

Costal
margin

Midline

Umbilicus

Anterosuperior
iliac spine

Poupart
ligament

Superior margin
of os pubis

(From Wilson and Giddens, 2009.)

Percussion Notes of the Abdomen

Note	Description	Location
Tympany	Musical note of higher pitch than resonance	Over air-filled viscera
Hyperresonance	Pitch lies between tympany and resonance	Base of left lung
Resonance	Sustained note of moderate pitch	Over lung tissue and sometimes over abdomen
Dullness	Short, high-pitched note with little resonance	Over solid organs adjacent to air-filled structures

Technique	Findings

Percuss abdomen

NOTE: **Percussion can be done independently or concurrently with palpation.**

- *Tone*
  Percuss in all four quadrants or nine regions.

  EXPECTED: Tympany predominant. Dullness over organs and solid masses. Dullness in suprapubic area from distended bladder. See table on p. 136 for percussion notes.
  UNEXPECTED: Dullness predominant.

- *Liver span*
  To determine lower liver border, percuss upward at right midclavicular line, as shown in figure on p. 138, and mark with a pen where tympany changes to dullness. To determine upper liver border, percuss downward at right midclavicular line from an area of lung resonance, and mark change to dullness. Measure the distance between marks to estimate vertical span.

  EXPECTED: Lower border usually begins at or slightly below costal margin. Upper border usually begins at fifth to seventh intercostal space. Span generally ranges from 6 to 12 cm in adults.
  UNEXPECTED: Lower liver border >2-3 cm below costal margin. Upper liver border above the fifth or below the seventh intercostal space. Span <6 cm or >12 cm.

- *Spleen*
  Percuss just posterior to midaxillary line on left, beginning at areas of lung resonance and moving in several directions. Percuss lowest intercostal space in left anterior axillary line before and after patient takes deep breath.

  EXPECTED: Small area of dullness from sixth to tenth rib. Tympany before and after deep breath.
  UNEXPECTED: Large area of dullness (check for full stomach or feces-filled intestine). Tone change from tympany to dullness with inspiration.

- *Stomach*
  Percuss in area of left lower anterior rib cage and left epigastric region.

  EXPECTED: Tympany of gastric air bubble (lower than intestine tympany).
  UNEXPECTED: Dullness.

ABDOMEN

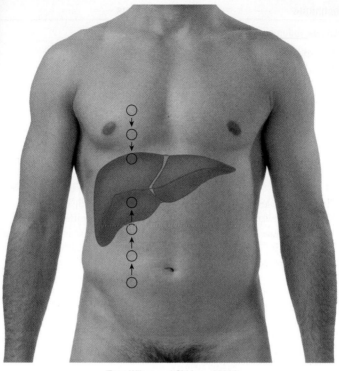

(From Wilson and Giddens, 2009.)

Technique	Findings
Lightly palpate abdomen Stand at patient's right side. Systematically palpate all quadrants, avoiding areas previously identified as problem spots. With palmar surface of fingers, depress abdominal wall up to 1 cm with light, even circular motion.	**EXPECTED:** Abdomen smooth with consistent softness. Possible tension from palpating too deeply, cold hands, or ticklishness. **UNEXPECTED:** Muscular tension or resistance, tenderness, or masses. If resistance is present, place pillow under patient's knees and ask patient to breathe slowly through mouth. Feel for relaxation of rectus abdominis muscles on expiration. Continuing tension signals involuntary response to localized or generalized rigidity.

Technique	Findings

Palpate abdomen with moderate pressure

Using same hand position as above, palpate all quadrants again, this time with moderate pressure.

EXPECTED: Soft, nontender
UNEXPECTED: Tenderness.

Deeply palpate abdomen

With same hand position as above, repeat palpation in all quadrants or regions, pressing deeply and evenly into abdominal wall. Move fingers back and forth over abdominal contents. Use bimanual technique—exerting pressure with top hand and concentrating on sensation with bottom hand, as shown in figure below—if obesity or muscular resistance makes deep palpation difficult. To help determine whether masses are superficial or intraabdominal, have patient lift head from examining table to contract abdominal muscles and obscure intraabdominal masses.

EXPECTED: Possible sensation of abdominal wall sliding back and forth. Possible awareness of borders of rectus abdominis muscles, aorta, and portions of colon. Possible tenderness over cecum, sigmoid colon, and aorta and in midline near xiphoid process.
UNEXPECTED: Bulges, masses, tenderness unrelated to deep palpation of cecum, sigmoid colon, aorta, xiphoid process. Note location, size, shape, consistency, tenderness, pulsation, mobility, movement (with respiration) of any masses.

ABDOMEN

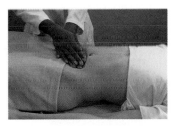

- *Umbilical ring and umbilicus*
  Palpate umbilical ring and around umbilicus. Note whether ring is incomplete or soft in center.

EXPECTED: Umbilical ring circular and free of irregularities. Umbilicus either slightly inverted or everted.
UNEXPECTED: Bulges, nodules, granulation. Protruding umbilicus.

ABDOMEN

Technique	Findings
• *Liver* Place left hand under patient at eleventh and twelfth ribs, lifting to elevate liver toward abdominal wall. Place right hand on abdomen, fingers extended toward head with tips on right midclavicular line below level of liver dullness, as shown in figure at right. Alternatively, place right hand parallel to right costal margin, as shown in bottom figure at right. Press right hand gently but deeply in and up. Ask patient to breathe comfortably a few times and then take a deep breath. Feel for liver edge as diaphragm pushes it down. If palpable, repeat maneuver medially and laterally to costal margin.	**EXPECTED:** Usually liver is not palpable. If felt, liver edge should be firm, smooth, even. **UNEXPECTED:** Tenderness, nodules, or irregularity. 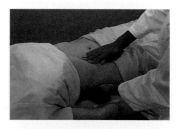 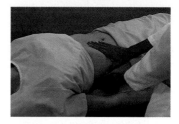
• *Gallbladder* Palpate below liver margin at lateral border of rectus abdominis muscle.	**EXPECTED:** Gallbladder not palpable. **UNEXPECTED:** Palpable, tender. If tender (possible cholecystitis), palpate deeply during inspiration and observe for pain (Murphy sign).

Technique	Findings
• *Spleen*	**EXPECTED:** Spleen usually not palpable by either method.
Still standing on right side, reach across patient with left hand, place it beneath patient over left costovertebral angle (CVA), and lift spleen anteriorly toward abdominal wall. As shown in figure at right, place right hand on abdomen below left costal margin and—using findings from percussion—gently press fingertips inward toward spleen while asking patient to take a deep breath. Feel for spleen as it moves downward toward fingers.	**UNEXPECTED:** Palpable spleen.

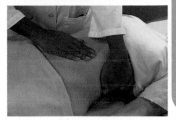

Repeat with patient lying on right side, as shown in bottom figure at right, with hips and knees flexed. Press inward with left hand while using fingertips of right hand to feel edge of spleen.

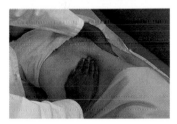

• *Left kidney*
Standing on patient's right, reach across with left hand, and place over left flank; then place right hand at patient's left costal margin. Ask patient to inhale deeply while you elevate left flank and palpate deeply with right hand.

EXPECTED: Left kidney usually not palpable.
UNEXPECTED: Tenderness.

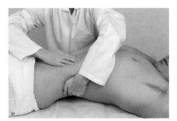

Technique	Findings
• *Right kidney* Standing on patient's right, place left hand under right flank, then place right hand at patient's right costal margin. Ask patient to inhale deeply while you elevate right flank and palpate deeply with right hand.	**EXPECTED:** If palpable, right kidney should be smooth and firm with rounded edges. **UNEXPECTED:** Tenderness. 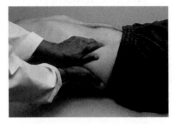
• *Aorta* Palpate deeply slightly to left of midline and feel for aortic pulsation. As an alternative technique, place palmar surface of hands with fingers extended on midline; press fingers deeply inward on each side of aorta and feel for pulsation. For thin patients, use one hand, placing thumb and fingers on either side of aorta.	**EXPECTED:** If prominent, pulsation should be anterior in direction. **UNEXPECTED:** Prominent lateral pulsation (suggests aortic aneurysm). 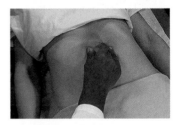
• *Urinary bladder* Percuss distended bladder to help determine outline, then palpate.	**EXPECTED:** Ordinarily not palpable unless distended with urine. If distended, bladder should be smooth, round, and tense, and on percussion will elicit lower note than surrounding air-filled intestines. **UNEXPECTED:** Palpable when not distended with urine.

Technique	Findings

With patient sitting, percuss CVAs
Stand behind patient. Right side: Place left hand over right CVA and strike with ulnar surface of right fist. Left side: Repeat with hands reversed.

EXPECTED: No tenderness.
UNEXPECTED: Kidney tenderness or pain.

Pain assessment
Keep eyes on patient's face while examining abdomen. To help characterize pain, have patient cough, take a deep breath, jump, or walk. Ask whether patient is hungry.

UNEXPECTED: Unwillingness to move, nausea, vomiting, areas of localized tenderness. Lack of hunger. See box and table on p. 144.

Iliopsoas muscle test
Use test for suspected appendicitis. With patient supine, place hand over right lower thigh. Ask patient to raise leg, flexing at hip, while you push downward.

UNEXPECTED: Right lower quadrant (RLQ) pain.

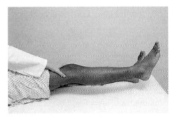

Obturator muscle test
Use test for suspected ruptured appendix or pelvic abscess. With patient supine, ask patient to flex right leg at hip and bend knee to 90 degrees. Hold leg just above knee, grasp ankle, and rotate leg laterally and medially, as shown in figure.

UNEXPECTED: Pain in right hypogastric region.

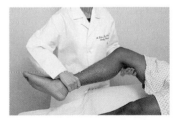

ABDOMEN

ABDOMEN

Some Causes of Pain Perceived in Anatomic Regions

Right Upper Quadrant
Duodenal ulcer
Hepatitis
Hepatomegaly
Lower lobe pneumonia
Cholecystitis

Right Lower Quadrant
Appendicitis
Salpingitis
Ovarian cyst
Tubo-ovarian abscess
Ruptured ectopic pregnancy
Renal/ureteral stone
Strangulated hernia
Meckel diverticulitis
Regional ileitis
Perforated cecum

Periumbilical
Intestinal obstruction
Acute pancreatitis
Early appendicitis

Periumbilical, cont'd
Mesenteric thrombosis
Aortic aneurysm
Diverticulitis

Left Upper Quadrant
Ruptured spleen
Gastric ulcer
Aortic aneurysm
Perforated colon
Lower lobe pneumonia

Left Lower Quadrant
Sigmoid diverticulitis
Salpingitis
Ovarian cyst
Ruptured ectopic pregnancy
Tubo-ovarian abscess
Renal/ureteral stone
Strangulated hernia
Perforated colon
Regional ileitis
Ulcerative colitis

Quality and Onset of Abdominal Pain

Characteristic	Possible Related Condition
Burning	Peptic ulcer
Cramping	Biliary colic, gastroenteritis
Colic	Appendicitis with impacted feces; renal stone
Aching	Appendiceal irritation
Knife-like	Pancreatitis
Ripping, tearing	Aortic dissection
Gradual onset	Infection
Sudden onset	Duodenal ulcer, acute pancreatitis, obstruction, perforation

AIDS TO DIFFERENTIAL DIAGNOSIS

Subjective Data	Objective Data

Hiatal Hernia with Esophagitis

Epigastric pain and/or heartburn that worsens with lying down and is relieved by sitting up or antacids; water brash (mouth fills with fluid); dysphagia; sudden onset of vomiting, pain, complete dysphagia are symptoms of hernia incarceration.

With severe disease, may have erythema of the posterior pharynx and edematous vocal cords.

Gastroesophageal Reflux Disease

Heartburn or acid indigestion (burning chest pain, located behind breastbone that moves up toward the neck and throat); sour taste of acid in the back of the throat or hoarseness; symptoms in infants and children include back arching or fussiness with feeding, regurgitation, and vomiting; can precipitate acute asthma exacerbation, can cause respiratory problems from aspiration, and can lead to esophageal bleeding.

With severe disease, may have erythema of the posterior pharynx and edematous vocal cords; when frequent emesis occurs, may cause failure to thrive in an infant.

Duodenal Ulcer

Localized epigastric pain that occurs when the stomach is empty and is relieved with food or antacids; with upper gastrointestinal bleeding, may have hematemesis, melena, dizziness, syncope.

Anterior wall ulcers may produce tenderness on palpation of the abdomen; with significant upper gastrointestinal bleeding, may have decreased blood pressure, increased pulse rate, and decreased hematocrit level; signs of an acute abdomen could indicate perforation of duodenum, **a life-threatening event.**

Subjective Data	Objective Data
Acute Diarrhea Abrupt onset, lasts <2 weeks; abdominal pain, diarrhea, nausea, vomiting, fever, tenesmus (feeling of incomplete defecation); if symptoms occur in two or more persons after ingestion of the same food, suspect food poisoning.	Diffuse abdominal tenderness; can mimic peritoneal inflammation with RLQ pain or guarding; when severe, may develop moderate to severe dehydration (decreased blood pressure, increased heart rate).
Crohn's Disease Chronic diarrhea (can be bloody) with malabsorption, cramping characterized by unpredictable flares and remissions.	Abdominal mass may be palpated from thickened or inflamed bowel; perianal skin tags, fistulae, and abscess formation; extraintestinal findings include arthritis of large joints, erythema nodosum, pyoderma gangrenosum.
Ulcerative Colitis Bloody, frequent (up to 20-30 stools/day), watery diarrhea; mild to severe symptoms based on degree of colon involvement; weight loss, fatigue, general debilitation.	Generally do not have fistulae or perianal disease; cholestatic pattern of elevated transaminases suggests sclerosing cholangitis.
Irritable Bowel Syndrome Cluster of symptoms consisting of abdominal pain, bloating, constipation, and diarrhea; some patients have alternating diarrhea and constipation; mucus may be present around or within the stool.	Generally unremarkable examination.
Colon Cancer May have abdominal pain, gross blood in stool, but more often presents with occult blood in stool on fecal occult blood test; may have change in frequency or character of stool.	With progressive disease, may have palpable mass in right (RLQ) or left lower quadrant (LLQ); rectal mass may be palpable on digital rectal examination.

Subjective Data	Objective Data

Hepatitis
Some asymptomatic; others experience jaundice, anorexia, abdominal pain, clay-colored stools, tea-colored urine, fatigue. | Abnormal liver function tests; jaundice; hepatomegaly.

Cirrhosis
Some asymptomatic; others experience jaundice, anorexia, abdominal pain, clay-colored stools, tea-colored urine, fatigue; may report prominent abdominal vasculature, cutaneous spider angiomas, hematemesis, abdominal fullness. | Abnormal liver function tests; jaundice; initially with firm, nontender enlarged liver; in severe disease, liver size decreases, portal hypertension and esophageal varices may develop, and muscle wasting and nutritional deficiencies may occur.

Cholecystitis
Acute: Right upper quadrant (RUQ) pain with radiation around midtorso to right scapular region; pain is abrupt and severe, lasting 2-4 hours; may have fever, jaundice, anorexia. *Chronic:* Repeated acute attacks; fat intolerance, flatulence, nausea, anorexia, nonspecific abdominal pain. | Marked tenderness in the RUQ or epigastrium; involuntary guarding or rebound tenderness; some with full palpable gallbladder in RUQ.

Chronic Pancreatitis
Unremitting abdominal pain, weight loss, steatorrhea. | Diffuse abdominal tenderness to palpation; involuntary guarding and abdominal distention can occur; elevated pancreatic enzymes (amylase and lipase); may develop pseudocyst formation; with advanced disease, may show subcutaneous fat and temporal wasting from malnutrition.

Pyelonephritis
Flank pain, dysuria, fever; may have rigors, urinary frequency, urgency, and hematuria. | Ill appearing with CVA tenderness; pyuria and bacteria.

ABDOMEN

Subjective Data	Objective Data
Renal Calculi	
Fever, dysuria, hematuria; severe cramping and flank pain with nausea and vomiting; as the stone passes, pain typically moves from flank to groin to scrotal or labial area.	Ill appearing with severe cramping pain; may have CVA tenderness or abdominal tenderness on palpation; microscopic hematuria.
Appendicitis	
Initially periumbilical or epigastric pain; colicky; later becomes localized to RLQ; anorexia, nausea, or vomiting after onset of pain; low-grade fever.	Guarding, tenderness, positive iliopsoas and/or obturator signs, RLQ pain on palpation (McBurney's sign).

Abdominal Signs Associated with Common Abnormal Conditions

Sign	Description	Associated Conditions
Aaron	Pain or distress occurs in the area of patient's heart or stomach on palpation of McBurney point	Appendicitis
Ballance	Fixed dullness to percussion in left flank and dullness in right flank that disappear on change of position	Peritoneal irritation
Blumberg	Rebound tenderness	Peritoneal irritation, appendicitis
Cullen	Ecchymosis around umbilicus	Hemoperitoneum, pancreatitis, ectopic pregnancy
Dance	Absence of bowel sounds in RLQ	Intussusception
Grey Turner	Ecchymosis of flanks	Hemoperitoneum, pancreatitis
Kehr	Abdominal pain radiating to left shoulder	Spleen rupture, renal calculi, ectopic pregnancy

Abdominal Signs Associated with Common Abnormal Conditions—cont'd

Sign	Description	Associated Conditions
Markle (heel jar)	Patient stands with straightened knees, then raises up on toes, relaxes, and allows heels to hit floor, thus jarring body; action will cause abdominal pain if positive	Peritoneal irritation, appendicitis
McBurney	Rebound tenderness and sharp pain when McBurney's point is palpated (⅔ the distance from the umbilicus to the anterior superior iliac spine)	Appendicitis
Murphy	Abrupt cessation of inspiration on palpation of gallbladder	Cholecystitis
Romberg-Howship	Pain down medial aspect of thigh to knees	Strangulated obturator hernia
Rovsing	RLQ pain intensified by left lower quadrant abdominal palpation	Peritoneal irritation, appendicitis

Conditions That Produce Acute Abdominal Pain

Condition	Usual Pain Characteristics	Possible Associated Findings
Appendicitis	Initially periumbilical or epigastric; colicky; later becomes localized to RLQ, often at McBurney's point	Guarding, tenderness; positive iliopsoas and positive obturator tests, RLQ skin hyperesthesia; anorexia, nausea, or vomiting after onset of pain; low-grade fever; positive Aaron, Rovsing, Markle, and McBurney signs*
Peritonitis	Onset sudden or gradual; pain generalized or localized, dull or severe and unrelenting; guarding; pain on deep inspiration	Shallow respiration; positive Blumberg, Markle, and Ballance signs; reduced bowel sounds, nausea and vomiting; positive obturator and iliopsoas tests

Continued

ABDOMEN

Conditions That Produce Acute Abdominal Pain—cont'd

Condition	Usual Pain Characteristics	Possible Associated Findings
Cholecystitis	Severe, unrelenting RUQ or epigastric pain; may be referred to right subscapular area	RUQ tenderness and rigidity, positive Murphy sign, palpable gallbladder, anorexia, vomiting, fever, possible jaundice
Pancreatitis	Dramatic, sudden, excruciating left upper quadrant (LUQ), epigastric, or umbilical pain; may be present in one or both flanks; may be referred to left shoulder	Epigastric tenderness, vomiting, fever, shock; positive Grey Turner sign; positive Cullen sign; both signs may occur 2-3 days after onset
Salpingitis	Lower quadrant, worse on left	Nausea, vomiting, fever, suprapubic tenderness, rigid abdomen, pain on pelvic examination
Pelvic inflammatory disease	Lower quadrant, increases with activity	Tender adnexa and cervix, cervical discharge, dyspareunia
Diverticulitis	Epigastric, radiating down left side of abdomen especially after eating; may be referred to back	Flatulence, borborygmi, diarrhea, dysuria, tenderness on palpation
Perforated gastric or duodenal ulcer	Abrupt RUQ; may be referred to shoulders	Abdominal free air and distention with increased resonance over liver; tenderness in epigastrium or RUQ; rigid abdominal wall, rebound tenderness
Intestinal obstruction	Abrupt, severe, spasmodic; referred to epigastrium, umbilicus	Distention, minimal rebound tenderness, vomiting, localized tenderness, visible peristalsis; bowel sounds absent (with paralytic obstruction) or hyperactive high-pitched (with mechanical obstruction)
Volvulus	Referred to hypogastrium and umbilicus	Distention, nausea, vomiting, guarding; sigmoid loop volvulus may be palpable

Conditions That Produce Acute Abdominal Pain—cont'd

Condition	Usual Pain Characteristics	Possible Associated Findings
Leaking abdominal aneurysm	Steady throbbing midline over aneurysm; may penetrate to back, flank	Nausea, vomiting, abdominal mass, bruit
Biliary stones, colic	Episodic, severe, RUQ, or epigastrium lasting 15 min to several hours; may be referred to subscapular area, especially right	RUQ tenderness, soft abdominal wall, anorexia, vomiting, jaundice, subnormal temperature
Renal calculi	Intense; flank, extending to groin and genitals; may be episodic	Fever, hematuria; positive Kehr sign
Ectopic pregnancy	Lower quadrant; referred to shoulder; with rupture is agonizing	Hypogastric tenderness, symptoms of pregnancy, spotting, irregular menses, soft abdominal wall, mass on bimanual pelvic examination; ruptured: shock, rigid abdominal wall, distention; positive Kehr, Cullen signs
Ruptured ovarian cyst	Lower quadrant, steady, increases with cough or motion	Vomiting, low-grade fever, anorexia, tenderness on pelvic examination
Splenic rupture	Intense; LUQ, radiating to left shoulder; may worsen with foot of bed elevated	Shock, pallor, lowered temperature

*See table on pp. 148-149 for explanation of signs.

Conditions That Produce Chronic Abdominal Pain

Condition	Usual Pain Characteristics	Possible Associated Findings
Irritable bowel syndrome	Hypogastric pain; crampy, variable, infrequent; associated with bowel function	Unremarkable physical examination; pain associated with gas, bloating, distention; relief with passage of flatus, feces

Continued

ABDOMEN

Conditions That Produce Chronic Abdominal Pain—cont'd

Condition	Usual Pain Characteristics	Possible Associated Findings
Lactose intolerance	Crampy pain after drinking milk or eating milk products	Associated diarrhea; unremarkable physical examination
Diverticular disease	Localized pain	Abdominal tenderness, fever
Constipation	Colicky or dull and steady pain that does not progress or worsen	Fecal mass palpable, stool in rectum
Uterine fibroids	Pain related to menses, intercourse	Palpable myoma(s)
Hernia	Localized pain that increases with exertion or lifting	Hernia on physical examination
Esophagitis/gastroesophageal reflux disease	Burning, gnawing pain in midepigastrium, worsens with recumbency	Unremarkable physical examination
Peptic ulcer	Burning or gnawing pain	May have epigastric tenderness on palpation
Gastritis	Constant burning pain in epigastrium	May be accompanied by nausea, vomiting, diarrhea, or fever; unremarkable physical examination

Modified from Dains et al, 2011. Advanced Health Assessment & Clinical Diagnosis in Primary Care (Mosby) – Trade paperback (2011) by Joyce E Dains, Linda Ciofu Baumann, Pamela Scheibel.

Differential Diagnosis of Urinary Incontinence

Condition	History	Physical Findings
Stress incontinence	Small-volume incontinence with coughing, sneezing, laughing, running; history of prior pelvic surgery	Pelvic floor relaxation; cystocele, rectocele; lax urethral sphincter; loss of urine with provocative testing; atrophic vaginitis; postvoid residual <100 mL

Differential Diagnosis of Urinary Incontinence—cont'd

Condition	History	Physical Findings
Urge incontinence	Uncontrolled urge to void; large-volume incontinence; history of central nervous system disorders such as stroke, multiple sclerosis, parkinsonism	Unexpected findings only as related to central nervous system disorder; postvoid residual <100 mL
Overflow incontinence	Small-volume incontinence, dribbling, hesitancy; in men, symptoms of enlarged prostate: nocturia, dribbling, hesitancy, decreased force and calibre of stream	Distended bladder; prostate hypertrophy; stool in rectum, fecal impaction; postvoid residual >100 mL
	In neurogenic bladder: history of bowel problems, spinal cord injury, or multiple sclerosis	Evidence of spinal cord disease or diabetic neuropathy; lax sphincter; gait disturbance
Functional incontinence	Change in mental status, impaired mobility, new environment	Impaired mental status; impaired mobility
	Medications: hypnotics, diuretics, anticholinergic agents, α-adrenergic agents, calcium channel blockers	Impaired mental status or unexpected findings only as related to other physical conditions

ABDOMEN

ABDOMEN

PEDIATRIC VARIATIONS

EXAMINATION

Technique	Findings

Inspect abdomen in all four quadrants

Infant's abdomen should be examined, if possible, during a time of relaxation and quiet. Sucking on a pacifier may help to relax infant. The parent's lap can serve as the best examining surface for toddlers through age 3 years.

Technique	Findings
• Contour/symmetry	**EXPECTED:** Until the age of 3 years, abdomen will protrude when standing. **UNEXPECTED:** Distension can indicate organ enlargement, fecal impaction, or abdominal mass.
• Surface motion	**EXPECTED:** Pulsation in epigastric area in newborns and infants. **UNEXPECTED:** Peristaltic waves associated with pyloric stenosis.
Percuss abdomen • Tone	**EXPECTED:** More tympany is present in infants than adults because of air swallowing during crying and feeding.
Lightly and deeply palpate abdomen • Umbilical ring	**EXPECTED:** Infants and children may have an umbilical hernia (typically close spontaneously by 1-2 years of age).
• Liver	**EXPECTED:** Liver may be palpable in young children 2-3 cm below costal margin.

Technique	Findings	
	Age	*Liver Span (cm)*
	6 mo	2.4-2.8
	12 mo	2.8-3.1
	24 mo	3.5-3.6
	3 yr	4.0
	4 yr	4.3-4.4
	5 yr	4.5-5.1
	6 yr	4.8-5.1
	8 yr	5.1-5.6
	10 yr	5.5-6.1

ABDOMEN

SAMPLE DOCUMENTATION

Subjective. A 11 year old woman describes a burning sensation in epigastric area and chest. Occurs after eating, especially with spicy foods. Lasts 1 to 2 hours and is worse when lying down. Sometimes causes bitter taste in mouth. Also feels bloated. Antacids do not relieve symptoms. Denies nausea/vomiting/diarrhea. No cough or shortness of breath.

Objective. Abdomen rounded and symmetric, with white striae adjacent to umbilicus in all quadrants. A well-healed, 5-cm, white surgical scar evident in RLQ. No areas of visible pulsations or peristalsis. Active bowel sounds audible. Percussion tones tympanic over epigastrium. Liver span 8 cm at right midclavicular line. On inspiration, liver edge firm, smooth, and nontender. No splenomegaly. Musculature soft and relaxed to light palpation. No masses or areas of tenderness to deep palpation. No CVA tenderness.

EQUIPMENT

- Lamp or light source
- Drapes
- Speculum
- Gloves
- Water-soluble lubricant
- Papanicolaou (Pap) smear/human papillomavirus (HPV) collection equipment
  - Collection device (wooden or plastic spatula; cervical brush or broom)
  - Glass slides and cytologic fixative or fluid collection media
- Other specimen collection equipment as needed:
  - Cotton swabs
  - Culture plates or media
  - DNA tests for organisms

EXAMINATION

Have patient in lithotomy position, draped for minimal exposure.

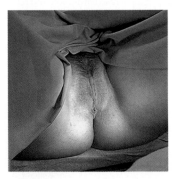

Technique	Findings

External Genitalia

Wash or sanitize hands and wear gloves on both hands

Ask patient to separate or drop open her knees. Tell patient you are beginning the examination, then touch lower thigh and—without breaking contact—move hand along thigh to external genitalia.

Inspect and palpate mons pubis

- *Characteristics*

  EXPECTED: Skin smooth and clean.
  UNEXPECTED: Improper hygiene.

- *Pubic hair*

  EXPECTED: Female pattern distribution.
  UNEXPECTED: Nits or lice.

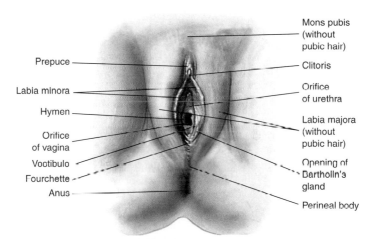

(From Lowdermilk and Perry, 2004.)

Inspect and palpate labia

- *Labia majora*

  EXPECTED: Gaping or closed, dry or moist, shriveled or full, tissue soft and homogeneous, usually symmetric.

Technique	Findings
	UNEXPECTED: Swelling, redness, tenderness, discoloration, varicosities, obvious stretching, or signs of trauma or scarring. If excoriation, rashes, or lesions are present, ask patient whether she has been scratching.
• *Labia minora* Separate labia majora with fingers of one hand. With other hand, palpate labia minora between thumb and second finger.	**EXPECTED:** Moist, dark pink inner surface. Tissue soft and homogeneous. **UNEXPECTED:** Tenderness, inflammation, irritation, excoriation, caking of discharge in tissue folds, discoloration, ulcers, vesicles, irregularities, or nodules. Hyperemia of fourchette not related to recent sexual activity.
Inspect clitoris	
• *Size and length*	**EXPECTED:** Length ≤2 cm; diameter 0.5 cm. **UNEXPECTED:** Enlargement, atrophy, inflammation, or adhesions.
Inspect urethral meatus and vaginal opening	
• *Urethral orifice*	**EXPECTED:** Slit or irregular opening, close to or in vaginal introitus, usually midline. **UNEXPECTED:** Discharge, polyps, caruncles, fistulas, lesions, irritation, inflammation, or dilation.
• *Vaginal introitus*	**EXPECTED:** Thin vertical slit or large orifice with irregular edges. Tissue moist. **UNEXPECTED:** Swelling, discoloration, discharge, lesions, fistulas, or fissures.

FEMALE GENITALIA

Technique	Findings

Milk Skene glands

Tell patient you will be inserting one finger into her vagina and pressing forward with it. With palm up, insert index finger to second joint, press upward, and milk Skene glands by moving finger outward. Perform on both sides of urethra and directly on urethra.

UNEXPECTED: Discharge or tenderness. Note color, consistency, odor of any discharge; obtain culture.

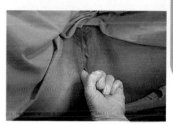

Palpate Bartholin glands

Tell patient she will feel you pressing around the entrance to her vagina. Palpate lateral tissue between index finger and thumb, then palpate entire area bilaterally, particularly posterolateral portion of labia majora.

EXPECTED: No swelling.
UNEXPECTED: Swelling, tenderness, masses, heat, fluctuation, or discharge. Note color, consistency, odor of any discharge; obtain culture.

Test vaginal muscle tone if indicated

Ask patient to squeeze vaginal opening around your finger.

EXPECTED: Fairly tight squeezing by some nulliparous women, less so by some multiparous women.
UNEXPECTED: Protrusion of cervix or uterus.

Locate the cervix

With your finger still in place, reach in farther to locate the cervix and note the direction in which it points. This may help you locate the cervix when you insert the speculum.

EXPECTED: Midline, may point horizontally, anteriorly, or posteriorly.
UNEXPECTED: Deviates to right or left.

Inspect for bulging and urinary incontinence if indicated

Ask patient to bear down.

EXPECTED: No bulging.
UNEXPECTED: Bulging of anterior or posterior wall, or urinary incontinence.

FEMALE GENITALIA

Technique	Findings

Inspect and palpate perineum

Compress perineal tissue between finger and thumb.

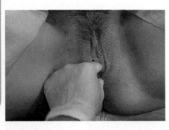

EXPECTED: Perineum surface smooth—generally thick and smooth in a nulliparous woman, thinner and rigid in a multiparous woman. Possible episiotomy scarring in women who have borne children.
UNEXPECTED: Tenderness, inflammation, fistulas, lesions, or growths.

Inspect anus
- *Skin characteristics*

EXPECTED: Skin darkly pigmented and possibly coarse.
UNEXPECTED: Scarring, lesions, inflammation, fissures, lumps, skin tags, or excoriation.

Internal Genitalia—Speculum Examination

If you touched the perineum or anal skin while examining the external genitalia, change gloves before beginning internal examination.

Lubricate speculum and gloved fingers with water or water-soluble gel lubricant. Water is preferred if obtaining a Pap smear.

Insert speculum
Tell patient she will feel you touching her again; then insert two fingers of hand not holding the speculum just inside vaginal introitus and gently press downward. Ask patient to breathe slowly and try to consciously relax her muscles.

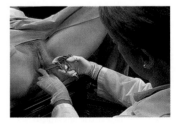

Use fingers of that hand to separate labia minora widely so that the vaginal opening becomes clearly visible. Then slowly insert speculum along path of least resistance, often slightly downward, avoiding trauma to urethra and vaginal walls. Some clinicians insert speculum blades at an oblique angle; others prefer to keep blades horizontal.

Technique	Findings

In either case, avoid touching clitoris, catching pubic hair, or pinching labial skin. Insert speculum the length of the vaginal canal. Maintaining downward pressure, open speculum by pressing on thumb piece. Sweep speculum slowly upward until cervix comes into view. Adjust light, then manipulate speculum farther into vagina to fully expose the cervix between anterior and posterior blades. Stabilize distal spread of blades and adjust proximal spread as needed.

Inspect cervix

• *Color*

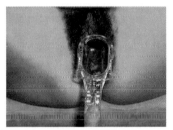

(From Edge and Miller, 1994.)

EXPECTED: Evenly distributed pink. Symmetric, circumscribed erythema around os can be expected.

UNEXPECTED: Bluish, pale, or reddened cervix (especially if patchy or with irregular borders)

• *Position*

EXPECTED: In midline, horizontal, or pointing anteriorly or posteriorly. Protruding into vagina 1-3 cm.

UNEXPECTED: Deviation to right or left. Protrusion into vagina >1-3 cm.

• *Size*

EXPECTED: 3 cm in diameter.
UNEXPECTED: >3 cm.

• *Shape*

EXPECTED: Uniform.
UNEXPECTED: Distorted.

Technique	Findings
• *Surface characteristics*	EXPECTED: Surface smooth. Possible symmetric, reddened circle around os (squamocolumnar epithelium). Possible small, white, or yellow raised round areas on cervix (nabothian cysts). UNEXPECTED: Friable tissue, red patchy areas, granular areas, or white patches.
• *Discharge* Note any discharge. Determine origin—cervix or vagina.	EXPECTED: Odorless; creamy or clear; thick, thin, or stringy (often heavier at midcycle or immediately before menstruation). UNEXPECTED: Odorous and white to yellow, green, or gray.
• *Size and shape of os* Follow standard precautions for safe collection of human secretions.	EXPECTED: Nulliparous woman: small, round, oval. Multiparous woman: usually a horizontal slit or irregular and stellate. UNEXPECTED: Slit resulting from trauma from induced abortion, difficult removal of intrauterine device, or sexual abuse.

Withdraw speculum and inspect vaginal walls

Unlock speculum and remove it slowly, rotating it so vaginal walls can be inspected. Maintain downward pressure and hook index finger over anterior blade as it is removed. Note odor of any discharge pooled in posterior blade, and obtain specimen if not already obtained.	EXPECTED: Vaginal wall color same pink as cervix or lighter; moist, smooth or rugated; and homogeneous. Thin, clear or cloudy, odorless secretions. UNEXPECTED: Reddened patches, lesions, pallor, cracks, bleeding, nodules, swelling. Secretions that are profuse; thick, curdy, or frothy; gray, green, or yellow; or malodorous.

Internal Genitalia—Bimanual Examination

Change gloves, then lubricate index and middle fingers of examining hand. Tell patient you are going to examine her internally with your fingers. Prevent thumb from touching clitoris during examination.

Obtaining Vaginal Smears and Cultures

Vaginal specimens are obtained while the speculum is in place in the vagina, but after the cervix and its surrounding tissue have been inspected. Collect specimens as indicated for a Pap smear, HPV testing, sexually transmitted infection screening, and wet mount. Label the specimen with the patient's name and a description of the specimen (e.g., cervical smear, vaginal smear, and culture). Be sure to follow standard precautions for the safe collection of human secretions.

Conventional Pap Smear

Brushes and brooms are now being used in conjunction with or instead of the conventional spatula to improve the quality of cells obtained. The cylindric-type brush (e.g., a Cytobrush) collects endocervical cells only. First, collect a sample from the ectocervix with a spatula. Insert the longer projection of the spatula into the cervical os. Rotate it 360 degrees, keeping it flush against the cervical tissue. Withdraw the spatula and spread the specimen on a glass slide. A single light stroke with each side of the spatula is sufficient to thin out the specimen over the slide. Fix the specimen and label as ectocervical. Then introduce the brush device into the vagina, and insert it into the cervical os until only the bristles closest to the handle are exposed. Slowly rotate one half to one full turn. Remove and prepare the slide. A single light stroke with each side of the spatula is sufficient to thin out the specimen over the slide. Fix the specimen and label as ectocervical. Then introduce the brush device into the vagina, and insert it into the cervical os until only the bristles closest to the handle are exposed. Slowly rotate one half to one full turn. Remove and prepare the endocervical smear by rolling the brush with moderate pressure across a glass slide. Fix the specimen and label as endocervical. Alternatively, both specimens can be placed on a single slide.

The broom-type brush is used for collecting ectocervical and endocervical cells at the same time. The broom has flexible plastic bristles, which are reported to cause less blood spotting after the examination. Introduce the brush into the vagina, and insert the central long bristles into the cervical os until the lateral bristles bend fully against the ectocervix. Maintain gentle pressure, and rotate the brush by rolling the handle between the thumb and forefinger three to five times to the left and right. Withdraw the brush and transfer the sample to a glass slide with two single "paint" strokes. Apply first one side of the bristle, then turn the brush over and paint the slide again in exactly the same area. Apply fixative and label as the ectocervical and endocervical specimen.

Liquid Pap Smear

For the liquid preparation technology, using the broom-type device, insert the central bristles of the broom into the endocervical canal deep enough to

Continued

allow the shorter bristles to fully contact the ectocervix. Push gently and then rotate the broom clockwise five times. Rinse the broom into the solution vial by pushing the broom into the bottom of the vial 10 times, forcing the bristles apart. As a final step, swirl the broom vigorously to further release material. Discard the collection device. Alternatively, deposit the broom end of the device directly into the collection vial. With any collection device, be sure to follow the manufacturer's and laboratory instructions to collect and preserve the specimen appropriately. Close the vial tightly to prevent leakage and loss of the sample during transport. The liquid sample is also used to test for HPV.

Gonococcal Culture Specimen

Immediately after the Pap smear is obtained, introduce a sterile cotton swab into the vagina and insert it into the cervical os. Hold it in place for 10 to 30 seconds. Withdraw the swab and spread the specimen in a large z pattern over the culture medium, rotating the swab at the same time. Label the tube or plate, and follow agency routine for transporting and warming the specimen. If indicated, an anal culture can be obtained after the vaginal speculum has been removed. Insert a fresh, sterile cotton swab about 2.5 cm into the rectum and rotate it in a full circle. Hold it in place for 10 to 30 seconds. Withdraw the swab, and prepare the specimen as described for the vaginal culture. Gonococcal cultures are now used less frequently than DNA testing for chlamydia and gonorrhea.

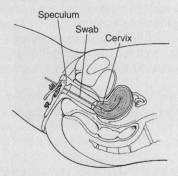

Speculum

Swab

Cervix

DNA Testing for Organisms

Use a Dacron swab (with a plastic or wire shaft) when collecting the specimen; wooden, cotton-tipped applicators may interfere with test results. Also be sure to check the expiration date so as not to use out-of-date materials. Insert the swab into the cervical os, and rotate the swab in the endocervical canal for 30 seconds to ensure adequate sampling and absorption by the swab. Avoid contact with the vaginal mucous membranes, which would contaminate the specimen. Remove the swab and place it in the tube containing the specimen reagent. Single- or dual-organism tests are available for *Chlamydia trachomatis* and *Neisseria gonorrhea.* Multiorganism tests are available for *Trichomonas vaginalis, Gardnerella vaginalis,* and *Candida* species

Wet Mount and Potassium Hydroxide Procedures

In a woman with vaginal discharge, these microscope examinations can demonstrate the presence of *T. vaginalis,* bacterial vaginosis, or candidiasis. For the wet mount, obtain a specimen of vaginal discharge using a swab. Smear the sample on a glass slide and add a drop of normal saline solution. Place a coverslip on the slide and view under the microscope. The presence of trichomonads indicates *T. vaginalis.* The presence of bacteria-filled epithelial cells (clue cells) indicates bacterial vaginosis. On a separate glass slide, place a specimen of vaginal discharge, apply a drop of aqueous 10% potassium hydroxide (KOH), and put a coverslip in place. The presence of a fishy odor (the "whiff test") suggests bacterial vaginosis. The KOH dissolves epithelial cells and debris, and facilitates visualization of the mycelia of a fungus. View under the microscope for the presence of mycelial fragments, hyphae, and budding yeast cells, which indicate candidiasis.

Technique	Findings
Palpate vaginal wall while inserting fingers into vagina	
Insert tips of index and middle fingers into vaginal opening and press downward, waiting for muscles to relax. Gradually insert fingers full length while palpating vaginal wall.	**EXPECTED:** Smooth and homogeneous. **UNEXPECTED:** Tenderness, lesions, cysts, nodules, masses, or growths.
Palpate cervix	
Locate cervix with palmar surface of fingers, feel end, and run fingers around circumference to feel fornices.	
• *Size, shape, length*	**EXPECTED:** Consistent with speculum examination.
• *Consistency*	**EXPECTED:** Firm in nonpregnant woman; softer in pregnant woman. **UNEXPECTED:** Nodules, hardness, or roughness.
• *Position*	**EXPECTED:** In midline horizontal or pointing anteriorly or posteriorly. Protruding into vagina 1-3 cm. **UNEXPECTED:** Deviation to right or left. Protrusion into vagina >1-3 cm.

Technique	Findings
• *Mobility* Grasp cervix gently between fingers and move from side to side. Observe patient's facial expression.	**EXPECTED:** 1- to 2-cm movement in each direction. Minimal discomfort. **UNEXPECTED:** Pain on movement ("cervical motion tenderness").
Palpate uterus • *Location and position* Place palmar surface of outside hand on abdominal midline, halfway between umbilicus and symphysis pubis, and place intravaginal fingers in anterior fornix. Slowly slide outside hand toward pubis while pressing down and forward with flat surface of fingers; at the same time, push inward and up with fingertips of intravaginal hand while pushing down on cervix with backs of fingers. If uterus is anteverted or anteflexed, you should feel fundus between fingers of two hands at level of pubis. If uterus cannot be felt with this maneuver, place intravaginal fingers together in posterior fornix and outside hand immediately above symphysis pubis. Press down firmly with outside hand while pressing inward against cervix with intravaginal hand. If uterus is retroverted or retroflexed, you should feel fundus. If uterus cannot be felt with either of these maneuvers, move intravaginal fingers to each side of cervix, and while keeping contact with cervix, press inward and feel as far as possible.	**EXPECTED:** In midline, horizontal, or pointing anteriorly or posteriorly. Protruding into vagina 1-3 cm. **UNEXPECTED:** Deviation to right or left. Protrusion into vagina >1-3 cm. 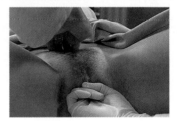

Technique	Findings

Slide fingers so they are on top and bottom of cervix, and continue pressing in while moving fingers to feel as much of uterus as possible (when uterus is in midposition, you will not be able to feel it with outside hand).

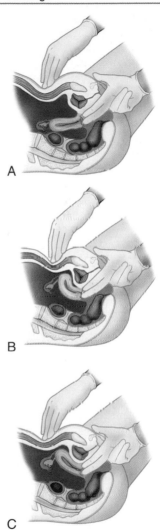

A

B

C

FEMALE GENITALIA

Technique	Findings

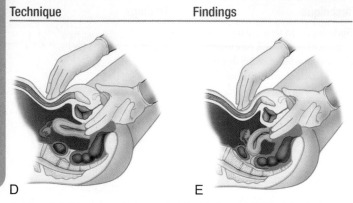

D   E

A, Anteverted. **B,** Anteflexed. **C,** Retroverted. **D,** Retroflexed. **E,** Midposition of uterus.

Technique	Findings
• *Size, shape, contour*	**EXPECTED:** Pear-shaped and 5.5-8 cm long (larger in all dimensions in multiparous women). Contour rounded and, in nonpregnant women, walls firm and smooth. **UNEXPECTED:** Larger than expected or interrupted contour or smoothness.
• *Mobility* Gently move uterus between intravaginal fingers and outside hand.	**EXPECTED:** Mobile in anteroposterior plane. **UNEXPECTED:** Fixed uterus or tenderness on movement.

Palpate ovaries

Place fingers of outside hand on lower right quadrant. With intravaginal hand facing up, place both fingers in right lateral fornix. Press intravaginal fingers deeply in and up toward abdominal hand, while sweeping flat surface of fingers of outside hand deeply in and obliquely down toward symphysis pubis. Palpate entire area by firmly pressing outside hand and intravaginal fingers together. Repeat on left side.

Technique	Findings
• *Consistency*	**EXPECTED:** If palpable, ovaries should feel firm, smooth, slightly to moderately tender. **UNEXPECTED:** Marked tenderness or nodularity. Palpable fallopian tubes.
• *Size*	**EXPECTED:** About 3 × 2 × 1 cm. **UNEXPECTED:** Enlargement.
• *Shape*	**EXPECTED:** Ovoid. **UNEXPECTED:** Distorted.
Palpate adnexal areas Use hand positions for palpating ovaries.	**EXPECTED:** Adnexa difficult to palpate. **UNEXPECTED:** Masses and tenderness. If adnexal masses are found, characterize by size, shape, location, consistency, tenderness.

Internal Genitalia—Rectovaginal Examination

Change gloves. This examination may be uncomfortable for the patient. Assure her that although she may feel the urgency of a bowel movement, she will not have one. Ask her to breathe slowly and try to relax her sphincter, rectum, and buttocks.

Insert index finger into vagina and middle finger into anus

To insert middle finger into anus, press against anus and ask patient to bear down. As she does, slip tip of finger into rectum just past sphincter.

Assess Sphincter Tone

Palpate area of anorectal junction and just above it. Ask patient to tighten and relax anal sphincter.	**EXPECTED:** Even sphincter tightening. **UNEXPECTED:** Extremely tight, lax, or absent sphincter.

Palpate Anterior Rectal Wall and Rectovaginal Septum

Slide both fingers in as far as possible, then ask patient to bear down. Rotate rectal finger to explore anterior rectal wall and palpate rectovaginal septum.	**EXPECTED:** Smooth and uninterrupted. Uterine body and uterine fundus sometimes felt with retroflexed uterus. **UNEXPECTED:** Masses, polyps, nodules, strictures, irregularities, tenderness.

FEMALE GENITALIA

Technique	Findings
Palpate posterior aspect of uterus Place outside hand just above symphysis pubis and press firmly and deeply down, while positioning intravaginal finger in posterior vaginal fornix and pressing strongly upward against posterior side of cervix, as shown in figure below. Palpate as much of posterior side of uterus as possible.	**EXPECTED:** Consistent with bimanual examination regarding location, position, size, shape, contour. **UNEXPECTED:** Tenderness.

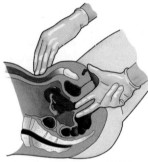

(From Lowdermilk and Perry, 2004.)

Palpate posterior rectal wall As you withdraw fingers, rotate intrarectal finger to evaluate posterior rectal wall.	**EXPECTED:** Smooth and uninterrupted. **UNEXPECTED:** Masses, polyps, nodules, strictures, irregularities, tenderness.
Note characteristics of feces when gloved finger removed	**EXPECTED:** Light to dark brown. **UNEXPECTED:** Blood. Note color and prepare specimen for fecal occult blood test if indicated.

Unless the patient is unable to, let patient wipe off the lubricating gel herself.

AIDS TO DIFFERENTIAL DIAGNOSIS

Subjective Data	Objective Data

Premenstrual Syndrome

Breast swelling and tenderness, acne, bloating and weight gain, headache or joint pain, food cravings, irritability, difficulty concentrating, mood swings, crying spells, depression. Symptoms occur 5-7 days before menses (luteal phase) and subside with onset of menses.

None; diagnosis based on symptoms.

Endometriosis

Pelvic pain, dysmenorrhea, heavy or prolonged menstrual flow.

May have no physical findings; on bimanual examination, tender nodules may be palpable along the uterosacral ligaments. Diagnosis confirmed by laparoscopy.

Condylomata Acuminata (genital warts)

Warty lesions on labia, within vestibule, or in perianal region.

Flesh-colored, whitish pink to reddish brown, discrete, soft growths on labia, vestibule, or perianal area; may occur singly or in clusters and may enlarge to cauliflower masses.

Genital Herpes

Painful lesions in genital area; history of sexual contact; may report burning or pain with urination.

Small, red vesicles in genital area.

Vaginal Infections

Vaginal discharge, possibly accompanied by urinary symptoms. Sometimes asymptomatic.

See table on pp. 173-174.

Cervical Carcinoma

Often asymptomatic; sometimes vaginal bleeding.

Hard granular surface at or near cervical os. Lesion can evolve to form extensive, irregular, easily bleeding cauliflower growth. Precancerous and early cancer changes detected by Pap smear, not by physical examination.

Subjective Data   Objective Data

Uterine Bleeding
See table on p. 175.

Terminology:

- Amenorrhea: absence of menstruation
- Polymenorrhea: shortened interval between periods—<19-21 days
- Oligomenorrhea: lengthened interval between periods—>35 days
- Hypermenorrhea: excessive flow during normal duration of regular periods
- Hypomenorrhea: decreased flow during normal duration of regular periods
- Menorrhagia: regular and normal interval between periods, excessive flow and duration
- Metrorrhagia: irregular interval between periods, excessive flow and duration
- Menometrorrhagia: irregular or excessive bleeding during periods and between periods

Pelvic Inflammatory Disease (PID)
Painful intercourse, painful urination, irregular menstrual bleeding, pain in the right upper abdomen.

Acute PID: Very tender bilateral adnexal areas. Chronic PID: Bilateral tender, irregular, fairly fixed adnexal areas.

Ovarian Cancer
Persistent and unexplained vague gastrointestinal symptoms such as generalized abdominal discomfort and/or pain, gas, indigestion, pressure, swelling, bloating, cramps, or feeling of fullness even after a light meal.

May have no physical findings; on bimanual examination, an enlarged ovary in premenopausal woman or a palpable ovary in postmenopausal women.

Differential Diagnosis of Vaginal Discharges and Infections

Condition	History	Physical Findings	Diagnostic Tests
Physiologic vaginitis	Increase in discharge; no foul odor, itching, or edema	Clear or mucoid discharge; pH <4.5	Wet mount: up to 3-5 white blood cells (WBCs); epithelial cells
Bacterial vaginosis (G. vaginalis)	Foul-smelling discharge; has concern about "fishy odor"	Homogeneous, thin, white or gray discharge; pH ≥4.5	Positive KOH "whiff" test; wet mount: positive clue cells
Candida vulvovaginitis (Candida albicans)	Pruritic discharge, itching of labia; itching may extend to thighs	White, curdy discharge; pH 4.0-5.0; cervix may be red; may have erythema of perineum and thighs	KOH prep: Mycelia, budding, branching yeast, pseudohyphae
Trichomoniasis (T. vaginalis)	Watery discharge; foul odor; dysuria and dyspareunia with severe infection	Profuse, frothy, greenish discharge; pH 5.0-6.6; red friable cervix with petechiae ("strawberry" cervix)	Wet mount: Round or pear-shaped protozoa, motile "gyrating" flagella
Gonorrhea (N. gonorrhoeae)	Partner with sexually transmitted disease; often asymptomatic or may have symptoms of PID	Purulent discharge from cervix; Skene/Bartholin gland inflammation; cervix and vulva may be inflamed	Gram stain, culture, DNA probe
Chlamydia (C. trachomatis)	Partner with nongonococcal urethritis often asymptomatic; may express concern about spotting after intercourse or urethritis	With or without purulent discharge; cervix may or may not be red or friable	DNA probe

Differential Diagnosis of Vaginal Discharges and Infections—cont'd

Condition	History	Physical Findings	Diagnostic Tests
Atrophic vaginitis	Dyspareunia; vaginal dryness; perimenopausal or postmenopausal	Pale, thin vaginal mucosa; pH >4.5	Wet mount: Folded, clumped epithelial cells
Allergic vaginitis	New bubble bath, soap, douche, or other hygiene products	Foul smell, erythema; pH <4.5	Wet mount: WBCs
Foreign body	Red and swollen vulva; vaginal discharge; history of tampon, condom, or diaphragm use	Bloody or foul-smelling discharge	Wet mount: WBCs

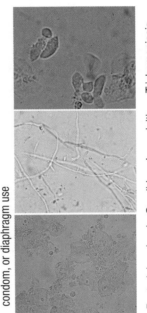

Bacterial vaginosis   Candida vulvovaginitis   Trichomoniasis

Types of Uterine Bleeding and Associated Causes

Type	Common Causes
Midcycle spotting	Midcycle estradiol fluctuation associated with ovulation
Delayed menstruation	Anovulation or threatened abortion with excessive bleeding
Frequent bleeding	Chronic PID, endometriosis, dysfunctional uterine bleeding (DUB), anovulation
Profuse menstrual bleeding	Endometrial polyps, DUB, adenomyosis, submucous leiomyomas, intrauterine device
Intermenstrual or irregular bleeding	Endometrial polyps, DUB, uterine or cervical cancer, oral contraceptives
Postmenopausal bleeding	Endometrial hyperplasia, estrogen therapy, endometrial cancer

FEMALE GENITALIA

PEDIATRIC VARIATIONS

EXAMINATION

Technique	Findings
Inspect external genitalia	
Examine infant using the frog-leg position.	**EXPECTED:** Genitalia of newborn reflect influence of maternal hormones. Labia majora and minora may be swollen, with labia minora often more prominent.
Inspect clitoris	
• *Size and length*	**EXPECTED:** The clitoris of a term infant is usually covered by labia minora and may appear relatively large.
Inspect urethral meatus and vaginal opening	
• *Inspect for discharge in infants and children*	**EXPECTED:** Mucoid whitish discharge is frequently seen during newborn period and sometimes as late as 4 weeks after birth. Discharge may be mixed with blood. **UNEXPECTED:** Mucoid discharge from irritation by diapers or powder; any discharge in children.

FEMALE GENITALIA

Technique	Findings

Assess pubertal development
Assess Tanner stages of female
pubic hair development.

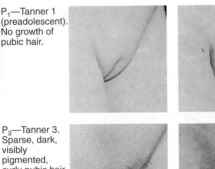

P₁—Tanner 1 (preadolescent). No growth of pubic hair.

P₂—Tanner 2. Initial, scarcely pigmented straight hair, especially along medial border of the labia.

P₃—Tanner 3. Sparse, dark, visibly pigmented, curly pubic hair on labia.

P₄—Tanner 4. Hair coarse and curly, abundant but less than adult.

P₅—Tanner 5. Lateral spreading; type and triangle spread of adult hair to medial surface of thighs.

P₆—Tanner 6. Further extension laterally, upward, or dispersed (occurs in only 10% of women).

Six stages of pubic hair development in females. *(Growth diagrams 1965 Netherlands: second national survey on 0-24-year-olds, by J. C. Van Wieringen, F. Wafelbakker, H. P. Verbrugge, J. H. DeHaas. Groningen: Noordhoff Uitgevers BV, The Netherlands.)*

"Red Flags" for Sexual Abuse

The following signs and symptoms in children or adolescents should raise your suspicion for sexual abuse. Remember, however, that any sign or symptom by itself is of limited significance; it may be related to sexual abuse, or it may be from another cause altogether. This is an area in which good clinical judgment is imperative. Each sign or symptom must be considered in context with the particular child's health status, stage of growth and development, and entire history.

Medical Concerns and Findings
- Evidence of general physical abuse or neglect
- Evidence of trauma and/or scarring in genital, anal, and perianal areas
- Unusual changes in skin color or pigmentation in genital or anal area
- Presence of sexually transmitted infection (oral, anal, genital)
- Anorectal problems such as itching, bleeding, pain, fecal incontinence, poor anal sphincter tone, bowel habit dysfunction
- Genitourinary problems such as rash or sores in genital area, vaginal odor or discharge, pain (including abdominal pain), itching, bleeding, discharge, dysuria, hematuria, urinary tract infections, enuresis

Examples of Nonspecific Behavioral Manifestations
- Problems with school
- Dramatic weight changes or eating disturbances
- Depression
- Anxiety
- Sleep problems or nightmares
- Sudden change in personality or behavior
- Increased aggression and impulsivity or destructiveness
- Sudden avoidance of certain people or places

Examples of Sexual Behaviors That Are Concerning
- Use of sexually provocative mannerisms
- Excessive masturbation or sexual behavior that cannot be redirected
- Age-inappropriate sexual knowledge or experience
- Repeated object insertion into vagina and/or anus
- Child asking to be touched/kissed in genital area
- Sex play between children with 4 or more years age difference
- Sex play that involves the use of force, threats, or bribes

Data from Hornor, 2004; Kellogg, 2005; Koop, 1988; and McClain et al, 2000.

Early Signs of Pregnancy

Following are physical signs that occur early in pregnancy. These signs, along with internal ballottement, palpation of fetal parts, and positive test results for urine or serum human chorionic gonadotropin, are probable indicators of pregnancy. They are considered "probable" because clinical conditions other than pregnancy may cause any one of them. Their occurrence together, however, creates a strong case for the presence of a pregnancy.

Sign	Finding	Approximate Weeks of Gestation
Goodell	Softening of cervix	4-6
Hegar	Softening of uterine isthmus	6-8
McDonald	Easy flexing of fundus on cervix	7-8
Braun von Fernwald	Fullness and softening of fundus near site of implantation	7-8
Piskacek	Palpable lateral bulge or soft prominence of one uterine cornu	7-8
Chadwick	Bluish color of cervix, vagina, vulva	8-12

SAMPLE DOCUMENTATION

Subjective. A 45-year-old woman with vaginal discharge and itching for past week. Has had yeast infections before. Completed course of antibiotics for sinusitis 2 days ago. Last menstrual period 2 weeks ago. Sexually active, one partner, mutually monogamous. No unusual vaginal bleeding. Does not douche.

Objective

External: Female hair distribution; no masses, lesions, or swelling. Urethral meatus intact without erythema or discharge. Perineum intact with healed episiotomy scar present. No lesions.

Internal: Vaginal mucosa pink and moist, rugated. No unusual odors. Profuse thick, white, curdy discharge. Cervix pink with horizontal slit midline; no lesions or discharge.

Bimanual: Cervix smooth, firm, mobile. No cervical motion tenderness. Uterus midline, anteverted, firm, smooth, nontender; not enlarged. Ovaries not palpable. No adnexal tenderness or masses.

Rectovaginal: Septum intact. Sphincter tone intact; anal ring smooth and intact. No masses or tenderness.

CHAPTER 16

Male Genitalia

EQUIPMENT

- Gloves
- Penlight

EXAMINATION

Have patient lying or standing to start examination.

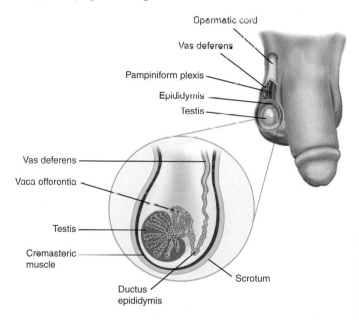

Spermatic cord

Vas deferens

Pampiniform plexis

Epididymis

Testis

Vas deferens

Vaca offorontia

Testis

Cremasteric muscle

Ductus epididymis

Scrotum

MALE GENITALIA

Technique	Findings
Wear gloves on both hands	
Inspect pubic hair	
• *Characteristics*	**EXPECTED:** Coarser than scalp hair.
• *Distribution*	**EXPECTED:** Male hair pattern distribution. Abundant in pubic region, continuing around scrotum to anal orifice, possibly continuing in narrowing midline to umbilicus. Penis without hair, scrotum with scant hair. **UNEXPECTED:** Alopecia.
Inspect glans penis	
• *Uncircumcised patient* Retract foreskin or ask patient to do so.	**EXPECTED:** Dorsal vein apparent. Foreskin easily retracted. White, cheesy smegma visible over glans. **UNEXPECTED:** Tight foreskin (phimosis). Lesions or discharge.
• *Circumcised patient*	**EXPECTED:** Dorsal vein apparent. Exposed glans erythematous and dry. **UNEXPECTED:** Lesions or discharge.
Examine external meatus of urethra (foreskin retracted in uncircumcised patient)	
• *Shape*	**EXPECTED:** Slit-like opening. **UNEXPECTED:** Pinpoint or round opening.
• *Location*	**EXPECTED:** On ventral surface and only millimeters from tip of glans. **UNEXPECTED:** Anyplace other than tip of glans or along shaft of penis.
• *Urethral orifice* Press glans between thumb and forefinger	**EXPECTED:** Opening glistening and pink. **UNEXPECTED:** Bright erythema or discharge.

Technique	Findings
Palpate penis Palpate the shaft of the penis.	**EXPECTED:** Soft (flaccid penis). **UNEXPECTED:** Tenderness, induration, or nodularity. Prolonged erection (priapism).
Strip urethra Firmly compress base of penis with thumb and forefinger; move toward glans.	**EXPECTYED:** No discharge **UNEXPECTED:** Discharge.

Inspect scrotum and ventral surface of penis

• *Color*	**EXPECTED:** Darker than body skin and often reddened in red-haired patients.
• *Texture*	**EXPECTED:** Surface possibly coarse. Small lumps on scrotal skin (sebaceous or epidermoid cysts) that sometimes discharge oily material.
• *Shape*	**EXPECTED:** Asymmetry. Thickness varying with temperature, age, emotional state. **UNEXPECTED:** Unusual thickening, often with pitting.

Palpate inguinal canal for direct or indirect hernia

With patient standing, ask him to bear down as if for bowel movement. While he strains, inspect area of inguinal canal and region of fossa ovalis. Ask patient to relax, and insert examining finger into lower part of scrotum and carry upward along vas deferens into inguinal canal, as shown in figure on p. 182. Ask patient to cough. Repeat examination on opposite side.	**EXPECTED:** Presence of oval external ring. **UNEXPECTED:** Feeling a viscus against examining finger with coughing. If hernia felt, note as indirect (felt within inguinal canal or even into scrotum) or direct (felt medial to external canal).

MALE GENITALIA

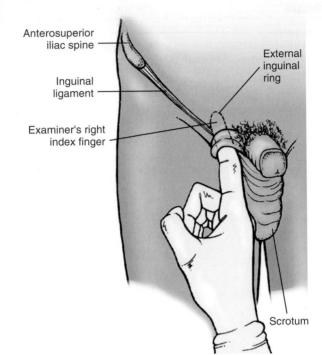

Labels: Anterosuperior iliac spine — Inguinal ligament — Examiner's right index finger — External inguinal ring — Scrotum

Technique	Findings
Palpate testes Use thumb and first two fingers. Compress gently.	
• *Descent*	**EXPECTED:** Both testes are present in scrotal sac **UNEXPECTED:** Cryptorchidism.
• *Consistency*	**EXPECTED:** Smooth and rubbery. Sensitive to gentle compression. **UNEXPECTED:** Tenderness or nodules. Total insensitivity to painful stimuli.
• *Texture*	**UNEXPECTED:** Irregular texture.
• *Size*	**UNEXPECTED:** Irregular size; asymmetry in size, <1 cm or >5 cm.

Technique	Findings
Palpate epididymides	
	EXPECTED: Smooth and discrete, with larger part cephalad. **UNEXPECTED:** Tenderness.
Palpate vas deferens Palpate from testicle to inguinal ring. Repeat with other testicle.	**EXPECTED:** Smooth and discrete. **UNEXPECTED:** Beaded or lumpy.
Palpate for inguinal lymph nodes Ask patient to lie supine, with knee slightly flexed on side of palpation.	**EXPECTED:** No palpable nodes. **UNEXPECTED:** Enlarged, tender, red or discolored, fixed, matted, inflamed, or warm nodes and increased vascularity.
Elicit cremasteric reflex bilaterally Stroke inner thigh with blunt instrument. Repeat with other thigh.	**EXPECTED:** The testicle and scrotum s rise on the stroked side **UNEXPECTED:** Absent reflex

MALE GENITALIA

AIDS TO DIFFERENTIAL DIAGNOSIS

Subjective Data	Objective Data

Hernia

See table on pp. 184-185.

Genital Herpes

Painful lesions on penis; sexually active; may report burning or pain with urination.

Superficial vesicles—located on glans, penile shaft, or base of penis; often associated with inguinal lymphadenopathy.

Condylomata Acuminata (genital warts)

Soft, painless, warty-like lesions on penis. Sexually active.

Single or multiple papular lesions; may be pearly, filiform, fungating (ulcerating and necrotic) cauliflower, or plaque-like.

Hydrocele

Painless enlargement or swelling of the scrotum.

Nontender, smooth, firm mass superior and anterior to the testis. Transilluminates.

Subjective Data	Objective Data
Varicocele	
Usually asymptomatic (and found during evaluation for infertility); may report scrotal pain or heaviness.	Abnormal tortuosity and dilated veins of pampiniform plexus within spermatic cord; described as "bag of worms."
Epididymitis	
Painful scrotum, urethral discharge, fever, pyuria, recent sexual activity.	Possible erythema of overlying scrotum, epididymis feels firm and lumpy, and may be slightly tender, and vasa deferentia may be beaded.
Testicular Torsion	
Acute onset of scrotal pain, often accompanied by nausea and vomiting; absence of systemic symptoms such as fever and myalgia.	Testicle is exquisitely tender; scrotal discoloration often present.
Testicular Cancer	
Painless mass in testicle, scrotal enlargement or swelling; sensation of heaviness in the scrotum, dull ache in the lower abdomen, back, or groin.	Irregular, nontender mass fixed on the testis; does not transilluminate.
Paraphimosis	
Retraction of the foreskin during penile examination, cleaning, urethral catheterization, or cystoscopy; penile pain and swelling.	Glans penis congested and enlarged; foreskin edematous; constricting band of tissue directly behind the head of the penis.

Distinguishing Characteristics of Hernias

	Indirect Inguinal	Direct Inguinal	Femoral
Incidence	Most common type of hernia; both sexes are affected; often patients are children and young males	Less common than indirect inguinal; occurs more in male than female individuals; more common in those older than 40 years	Least common type of hernia; occurs more often in female than male individuals; rare in children

	Indirect Inguinal	Direct Inguinal	Femoral
Pathway	Through internal inguinal ring; can remain in canal, exit external ring, or pass into scrotum; may be bilateral	Through femoral external inguinal ring; located in region of Hesselbach triangle; rarely enters scrotum	Through femoral ring, femoral canal, fossa ovalis
Presentation	Soft swelling in area of internal ring; pain on straining; hernia comes down canal and touches fingertip on examination	Bulge in area of Hesselbach triangle; usually painless; easily reduced; hernia bulges anteriorly, pushes against side of finger on examination	Right side presentation more common than left; pain may be severe; inguinal canal empty on examination

MALE GENITALIA

PEDIATRIC VARIATIONS

EXAMINATION

Technique	Findings
Inspect glans penis • *Uncircumcised patient* Retract foreskin.	**EXPECTED:** In children, foreskin is fully retractable by age 3–4 years. Before that age, forced retraction of foreskin may result in injury.
Palpate scrotum • *Descent* Palpate testes in children to determine whether testes have descended. If any mass other than testicles or spermatic cord is palpated in scrotum, determine whether it is filled with fluid, gas, or solid material.	**EXPECTED:** Bilaterally palpable; 1 cm. Considered descended if testis can be pushed into scrotum. **UNEXPECTED:** If penlight transilluminates, most likely contains fluid (hydrocele). If no light transillumination, most likely a hernia.

MALE GENITALIA

Technique	Findings
Evaluate maturation in adolescence	
Assess stage of pubertal development In boys, assess the stage of genital and pubic hair development.	**EXPECTED:** Tanner stages of male pubic hair and external genital development progress in the sequence shown on pp. 186-187. **UNEXPECTED:** Failure to mature and premature maturation.

G_1—Tanner 1. Testes, scrotum, and penis are the same size and shape as in the young child.

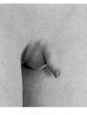

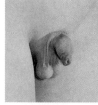

G_2—Tanner 2. Enlargement of scrotum and testes. The skin of the scrotum becomes redder, thinner, and wrinkled. Penis no larger or scarcely so.

G_3—Tanner 3. Enlargement of the penis, especially in length; further enlargement of testes; descent of scrotum.

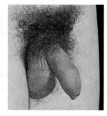

G_4—Tanner 4. Continued enlargement of the penis and sculpturing of the glans; increased pigmentation of scrotum.

G_5—Tanner 5 (adult stage). Scrotum ample, penis reaching nearly to bottom of scrotum.

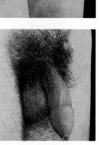

Five stages of penis and testes/scrotum development in males. *(Growth diagrams 1965 Netherlands: second national survey on 0-24-year-olds, by J. C. Van Wieringen, F. Wafelbakker, H. P. Verbrugge, J. H. DeHaas. Groningen: Noordhoff Uitgevers BV, The Netherlands.)*

P₁—Tanner 1 (preadolescent). No growth of pubic hair; that is, hair in pubic area no different from that on the rest of the abdomen.

P₂—Tanner 2. Slightly pigmented, longer, straight hair, often still downy; usually at base of penis, sometimes on scrotum. Stage is difficult to photograph.

P₃—Tanner 3. Dark, definitely pigmented, curly pubic hair around base of penis. Stage 3 can be photographed.

P₄—Tanner 4. Pubic hair definitely adult in type but not in extent (no further than inguinal fold).

P₅—Tanner 5 (adult distribution). Hair spread to medial surface of thighs, but not upward.

P₆—Hair spread along linea alba (occurs in 80% of men).

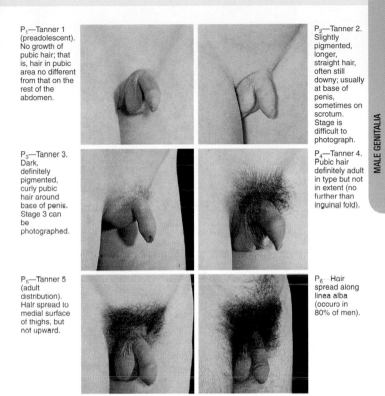

Six stages of pubic hair development in males. *(Growth diagrams 1965 Netherlands: second national survey on 0-24-year-olds, by J. C. Van Wieringen, F. Wafelbakker, H. P. Verbrugge, J. H. DeHaas. Groningen: Noordhoff Uitgevers BV, The Netherlands.)*

SAMPLE DOCUMENTATION

Subjective. Thirty-seven-year-old man reports painful burning lesions on his penis. Present past few days. Is sexually active. No burning on urination.

Objective. Hair in male pattern distribution. Circumcised glans without lesions or discharge. Urethral meatus patent on ventral surface at tip of glans. No urethral discharges. Penile shaft with vesicles present. Testes descended bilaterally; smooth without nodularity. Scrotal contents smooth without tenderness. Inguinal areas without bulges or hernias. Inguinal nodes palpable bilaterally. Cremasteric reflex elicited.

CHAPTER 17

Anus, Rectum, and Prostate

EQUIPMENT

- Gloves
- Water-soluble lubricant
- Light source
- Drapes
- Fecal occult blood testing materials if indicated

EXAMINATION

Have patient in knee-chest or left lateral position with hips and knees flexed, or standing with hips flexed and upper body supported by examining table. *Females:* Examination usually performed with patient in lithotomy position. Drape patient appropriately.

Technique	Findings
Wear gloves on both hands	
Inspect and palpate sacrococcygeal and perianal area	
• *Skin characteristics*	**EXPECTED:** Smooth and uninterrupted. **UNEXPECTED:** Lumps, rashes, tenderness, inflammation, excoriation, pilonidal dimpling, or tufts of hair.
Inspect anus Spread patient's buttocks. Examine, using penlight or lamp if needed, with patient relaxed, as well as with patient bearing down.	
• *Skin characteristics*	**EXPECTED:** Skin coarser and darker than on buttocks. **UNEXPECTED:** Skin lesions, skin tags or warts, external or internal hemorrhoids, fissures and fistulas, rectal prolapse, or polyps.

Technique	Findings

Inspect, palpate, assess sphincter tone

Put water-soluble lubricant on index or middle finger; press pad against anal opening, and ask patient to bear down to relax external sphincter. As relaxation occurs, slip tip of finger into anal canal, as shown in figure below. (Assure patient that although he or she may feel the urgency of a bowel movement, it will not occur.) Ask patient to tighten external sphincter around finger.

EXPECTED: Even sphincter tightening.
UNEXPECTED: Patient discomfort. Lax or extremely tight sphincter, tenderness.

Palpate muscular anal ring

Rotate finger.

EXPECTED: Smooth, even with consistent pressure exerted.
UNEXPECTED: Nodules or other irregularities.

Palpate lateral and posterior rectal walls

Insert finger farther and rotate to palpate lateral, then posterior, rectal walls. If helpful, perform bidigital palpation with thumb and finger by lightly pressing thumb against perianal tissue and bringing finger toward thumb.

EXPECTED: Smooth, even, uninterrupted.
UNEXPECTED: Nodules, masses, polyps, tenderness, or irregularities. (Internal hemorrhoids not ordinarily felt unless thrombosed.)

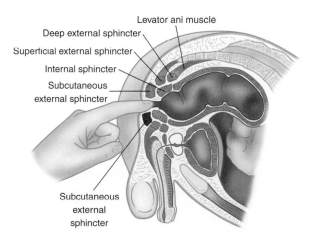

Levator ani muscle
Deep external sphincter
Superficial external sphincter
Internal sphincter
Subcutaneous external sphincter

Subcutaneous external sphincter

ANUS, RECTUM, AND PROSTATE

ANUS, RECTUM, AND PROSTATE

Technique	Findings
Males: Palpate posterior surface of prostate gland through anterior rectal wall	
Rotate finger and palpate anterior rectal wall and posterior surface of prostate gland. Alert patient that he may feel urge to urinate but will not.	
• *Consistency and characteristics of anterior rectal wall*	**EXPECTED:** Smooth, even, uninterrupted. **UNEXPECTED:** Nodules, masses, polyps, tenderness, or irregularities.
• *Consistency, contour, characteristics of prostate*	**EXPECTED:** Surface firm and smooth, lateral lobes symmetric, median sulcus palpable, seminal vesicles not palpable. **UNEXPECTED:** Rubberiness, bogginess, fluctuant softness, stony hard nodularity, tenderness, obliterated sulcus, or palpable seminal vesicles.
• *Mobility of prostate gland*	**EXPECTED:** Slightly movable.
• *Size of prostate gland*	**EXPECTED:** 4-cm diameter with <1 cm protruding into rectum. **UNEXPECTED:** Protrusion >1 cm (note distance of protrusion). Discharge that appears at urethral meatus (collect specimen for microscopic examination).
Females: Palpate uterus through anterior rectal wall	
Attempt to palpate uterus and cervix through anterior rectal wall.	
• *Position*	**EXPECTED:** Midline, retroflexed or retroverted. **UNEXPECTED:** Deviation to right or left.
• *Surface characteristics*	**EXPECTED:** Smooth. **UNEXPECTED:** Irregular.
Have patient bear down, and palpate deeper	
Ask patient to bear down while you reach farther into rectum. *Females:* Explore in cul-de-sac. *Males:* Explore above prostate.	**UNEXPECTED:** Tenderness of peritoneal area or nodules.

Technique	Findings
Withdraw finger and examine fecal material	
• *Color and consistency*	**EXPECTED:** Soft and brown. **UNEXPECTED:** Blood; pus; or light tan, gray, or tarry black stool. If indicated, fecal material can be tested for blood using a chemical guaiac procedure.

AIDS TO DIFFERENTIAL DIAGNOSIS

Subjective Data	Objective Data
Anal Warts (condyloma acuminata)	
Growths on the anus and genitalia.	Single or multiple papular lesions may be pearly, filiform, fungating (ulcerating and necrotic) cauliflower, or plaque-like.
Perianal and Perirectal Abscesses	
Pain and tenderness in anal area.	Tender, swollen, fluctuant mass; may be draining.
Enterobius Infestation in Children	
Intense perianal itching, especially at night.	Positive tape test. Press the sticky side of cellulose tape against the perianal folds and then press the tape on a glass slide. Nematodes can be seen on microscopic examination.
Anorectal Fissure	
Hard stools; pain, itching, bleeding.	Fissure most often in the posterior midline spastic internal sphincter.
Anorectal Fistula	
Chills, fever, nausea, vomiting, and malaise.	Elevated, red, granular tissue at external opening, possibly with serosanguineous or purulent drainage on compression of the area; palpable indurated tract.
Hemorrhoids	
Itching and bleeding; discomfort.	May or may not be visible; may be palpable as soft swellings. Thrombosed hemorrhoids appear as blue, shiny masses at anus.

Subjective Data	Objective Data
Rectal Carcinoma	
Bleeding; may be asymptomatic.	Sessile polypoid mass with nodular raised edges and areas of ulceration; consistency often stony, with irregular contour.
Prostatic Carcinoma	
Early carcinoma asymptomatic; symptoms of urinary obstruction as carcinoma advances.	Hard, irregular nodule may be palpable on prostate examination; prostate asymmetric, median sulcus may be obliterated; biopsy required for diagnosis.
Prostatitis	
Acute: Pain, urination problems, sexual dysfunction, fever, chills, shakes. *Chronic:* Asymptomatic, frequent bladder infections, frequent urination, persistent pain in the lower abdomen or back.	*Acute:* Prostate enlarged, acutely tender, and often asymmetric. May have urethral discharge and fever; bacteria in the urine. *Chronic:* Prostate boggy, enlarged, and tender or have palpable areas of fibrosis.
Benign Prostatic Hypertrophy	
Symptoms of urinary obstruction: hesitancy, decreased force and caliber of stream, dribbling, incomplete emptying of the bladder, frequency, urgency, nocturia, and dysuria.	Prostate smooth, rubbery, symmetric, and enlarged; median sulcus may or may not be obliterated.

Prostate Enlargement

Prostate enlargement is classified by the amount of protrusion into the rectum:

    Grade I: 1–2 cm

    Grade II: 2–3 cm

    Grade III: 3–4 cm

    Grade IV: >4 cm

PEDIATRIC VARIATIONS

EXAMINATION

Technique	Findings
Examine the patency of the anus and its position in all newborn infants. To determine patency, insert a lubricated catheter no more than 1 cm into the rectum. Inspect perianal area.	EXPECTED: Catheter inserts; patency confirmed by passage of meconium. UNEXPECTED: Not able to insert catheter; no evidence of stool. UNEXPECTED: Parental concerns about infant's or child's irritability at night or evidence that child has itching in perianal area may indicate presence of parasites such as roundworms or pinworms. Specimen collection and microscopic examination are necessary to confirm findings. Shrunken buttocks suggest a chronic debilitating disease. Asymmetric creases occur with congenital dislocation of the hips. Perirectal redness and irritation are suggestive of pinworms, *Candida*, or other irritants of the diaper area. Rectal prolapse results from constipation, diarrhea, or sometimes severe coughing or straining. Hemorrhoids are rare in children, and their presence suggests a serious underlying problem such as portal hypertension. Small, flat flaps of skin around the rectum (condylomata) may be syphilitic in origin. Sinuses, tufts of hair, and dimpling in the pilonidal area may indicate lower spinal deformities.

SAMPLE DOCUMENTATION

Subjective. A 57-year-old man is concerned about nighttime urination for the past several months, at least twice per night. Restricts fluid intake after 8 PM. Notices difficulty in starting stream. No pain or bleeding on urination. No change in caliber of stream. Denies change in bowel habits or stool characteristics. No history of prostatitis or enlarged prostate.

Objective. Perianal area intact without lesions or visible hemorrhoids. An external skin tag is visible in the 6 o'clock position. No fissures or fistulas. Sphincter tightens evenly. Prostate is symmetric, smooth, boggy, with 1-cm protrusion into rectum. Median sulcus present. Nontender, no nodules. Rectal walls free of masses. Moderate amount of soft brown stool present.

CHAPTER 18

Musculoskeletal System

EQUIPMENT

- Goniometer
- Skin-marking pencil
- Reflex hammer
- Tape measure

EXAMINATION

Begin examination as patient enters rooms, observing gait and posture. During examination, note ease of movement when patient walks, sits, rises, takes off garments, and responds to directions.

Technique	Findings

Posture and General Guidelines

Inspect skeleton and extremities, comparing sides

Inspect anterior, posterior, lateral aspects of posture; ability to stand erect; body parts; extremities.

- *Size, alignment, contour, symmetry*
  Measure extremities when lack of symmetry is noted in length or circumference.

EXPECTED: Bilateral symmetry of length, circumference, alignment, position and number of skinfolds, symmetric body parts; and aligned extremities.
UNEXPECTED: Gross deformity, lordosis, kyphosis, scoliosis, bony enlargement.

Inspect skin and subcutaneous tissues over muscles, cartilage, bones, joints

UNEXPECTED: Discoloration, swelling, or masses.

Inspect muscles and compare sides
- *Size and symmetry*

EXPECTED: Approximately symmetric bilateral muscle size.
UNEXPECTED: Gross hypertrophy or atrophy, fasciculations, or spasms.

MUSCULOSKELETAL SYSTEM

Technique	Findings

Palpate all bones, joints, surrounding muscles (palpate inflamed joints last)

- *Muscle tone*

EXPECTED: Firm.
UNEXPECTED: Hard or doughy, spasticity.

- *Characteristics*

UNEXPECTED: Heat, tenderness, swelling, fluctuation of a joint, synovial thickening, crepitus, resistance to pressure, or discomfort to pressure on bones and joints.

Test each major joint and related muscle groups for active and passive range of motion, and compare sides

Ask patient to move each joint through range of motion (see instructions for specific joints and muscles in individual sections that follow), then ask patient to relax as you passively move same joints until end of range is felt.

EXPECTED: Passive range of motion often exceeds active range of motion by 5 degrees. Range of motion with passive and active maneuvers should be equal between contralateral joints.
UNEXPECTED: Pain, limitation of motion, spastic movement, joint instability, deformity, contracture, discrepancies greater than 5 degrees between active and passive range of motion. When increase or limitation in range of motion is found, measure angles of greatest flexion and extension with goniometer, as shown in figure below, and compare with values as described for specific joints in individual extremities.

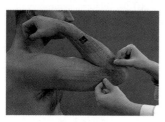

Goniometer.

Test major muscle groups for strength, and compare contralateral sides

For each muscle group, ask patient to contract a muscle by flexing or extending a joint and to resist as you apply opposing force. Compare bilaterally.

EXPECTED: Bilaterally symmetric strength with full resistance to opposition.
UNEXPECTED: Inability to produce full resistance. Grade muscular strength according to the following table.

Muscle Strength Assessment

Muscle Function Level	Grade
No evidence of contractility	0
Slight contractility, no movement	1
Full range of motion, gravity eliminated*	2
Full range of motion against gravity	3
Full range of motion against gravity, some resistance	4
Full range of motion against gravity, full resistance	5

*Passive movement.
(From Jacobson RD: Approach to the child with weakness and clumsiness, Pediatr Clin North Am 45[1]:145-168. 1998.)

Technique	Findings

Hands and Wrists

Inspect dorsum and palm of each hand

- *Characteristics and contour*

  EXPECTED: Palmar and phalangeal creases, palmar surfaces with central depression with prominent, rounded mound on thumb side (thenar eminence) and less prominent hypothenar eminence on little-finger side.

- *Position*

  EXPECTED: Fingers able to fully extend and align with forearm when in close approximation to each other.
  UNEXPECTED: Deviation of fingers to ulnar side or inability to fully extend fingers; swan neck or boutonnière deformities.

- *Shape*

  EXPECTED: Lateral finger surfaces gradually tapered from proximal to distal aspects.
  UNEXPECTED: Spindle-shaped fingers, bony overgrowths at phalangeal joints.

Palpate each joint in hand and wrist

Palpate interphalangeal joints with thumb and index finger, as shown in figure on p. 198, panel *A*; metacarpophalangeal joints with both thumbs, as shown in figure on p. 198, panel *B*; and wrist and radiocarpal groove with thumbs on dorsal surface and fingers on palmar aspect of wrist, as shown in figure on p. 198, panel *C*.

EXPECTED: Joint surfaces smooth.
UNEXPECTED: Nodules, swelling, bogginess, tenderness, or ganglion.

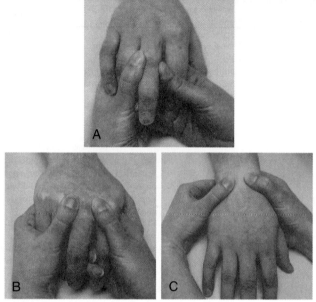

A, Palpating the interphalangeal joints with thumb and index finger. **B,** Palpating metacarpophalangeal joints with both thumbs. **C,** Palpating radiocarpal groove with thumbs on dorsal surface and fingers on palmar aspect of wrist.

Technique	Findings
Assess integrity of median nerve	
• *Tinel sign*	**UNEXPECTED:** Tingling sensation radiating from wrist to hand along pathway of median nerve.
Strike median nerve where it passes through carpal tunnel with index or middle finger.	
• *Thumb abduction test*	**EXPECTED:** Full resistance to pressure.
Apply downward pressure on thumb as patient holds thumb perpendicular to hand, palm side up.	**UNEXPECTED:** Inability to produce full resistance.
• *Phalen test*	**UNEXPECTED:** Numbness, paresthesia in distribution of median nerve.
Have patient hold both wrists in fully palmar-flexed position with dorsal surfaces pressed together for 1 minute.	

Technique	Findings
• *Katz hand diagram* Have patient mark specific locations of pain, numbness, tingling in hands and arms on diagram.	**UNEXPECTED:** Pain, numbness, tingling in pattern shown in figure below.

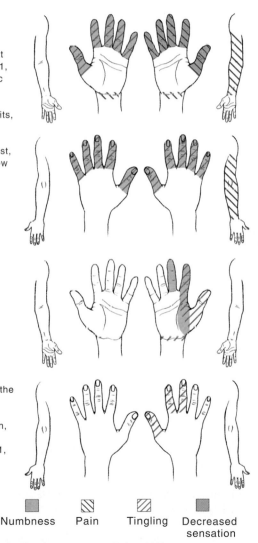

Classic pattern
Symptoms affect at least two of digits 1, 2, or 3. The classic pattern permits symptoms in the fourth and fifth digits, wrist pain, and radiation of pain proximal to the wrist, but it does not allow symptoms on the palm or dorsum of the hand.

Probable pattern
Same symptom pattern as classic except palmar symptoms are allowed unless confined solely to the ulnar aspect.
In the **possible pattern,** not shown, symptoms involve only one of digits 1, 2, or 3.

Numbness   Pain   Tingling   Decreased sensation

Redrawn from D'Arcy and McGee, 2000.

Technique	Findings
Test range of motion Ask patient to perform the following movements:	
• *Metacarpophalangeal flexion and hyperextension* Bend fingers forward at metacarpophalangeal joint, then stretch fingers up and back at knuckle.	**EXPECTED:** 90-degree metacarpophalangeal flexion and as much as 30-degree hyperextension.
• *Thumb opposition* Touch thumb to each fingertip and to base of little finger, then make a fist.	**EXPECTED:** Able to perform all movements.
• *Finger abduction and adduction* Spread fingers apart and then touch them together.	**EXPECTED:** Both movements possible.
• *Wrist extension and hyperextension* Bend hand at wrist up and down.	**EXPECTED:** 90-degree flexion and 70-degree hyperextension.
• *Radial and ulnar motion* With palm side down, turn each hand to right and left.	**EXPECTED:** 20-degree radial motion and 55-degree ulnar motion.
Test muscle strength Ask patient to perform the following movements:	
• *Wrist extension and hyperextension* Maintain wrist flexion while you apply opposing force.	**EXPECTED:** Bilaterally symmetric with full resistance to opposition. **UNEXPECTED:** Inability to produce full resistance.
• *Hand strength* Grip two of your fingers tightly.	**EXPECTED:** Firm, sustained grip. **UNEXPECTED:** Weakness or pain.
Elbows	
Inspect elbows in flexed and extended positions	
• *Contour*	**UNEXPECTED:** Subcutaneous nodules along pressure points of extensor surface of ulna.
• *Carrying angle* Inspect with arms at sides passively extended, palms facing forward.	**EXPECTED:** Usually 5 to 15 degrees laterally. **UNEXPECTED:** Lateral angle exceeding 15 degrees (cubitus valgus) or a medial carrying angle (cubitus varus).

Technique	Findings

Palpate extensor surface of ulna, olecranon process, medial and lateral epicondyles of humerus, groove on each side of olecranon process

Palpate with patient's elbow flexed at 70 degrees.

UNEXPECTED: Boggy, soft, tenderness at lateral epicondyle or along grooves of olecranon process and epicondyles.

Test range of motion

Ask patient to perform the following movements:

- *Flexion and extension*
Bend and straighten elbow.

EXPECTED: 160-degree flexion from full extension at 0 degrees.

- *Pronation and supination*
With elbow flexed at right angle, rotate hand from palm side down to palm side up.

EXPECTED: 90-degree pronation and 90-degree supination.
UNEXPECTED: Increased pain with pronation and supination of elbow.

Test muscle strength

Ask patient to maintain flexion and extension, as well as pronation and supination, while you apply opposing force.

EXPECTED: Bilaterally symmetric with full resistance to opposition.
UNEXPECTED: Inability to produce full resistance.

Shoulders

Inspect shoulders, shoulder girdle, clavicles and scapulae, area muscles

- *Size and contour*

EXPECTED: All shoulder structures symmetric in size and contour.
UNEXPECTED: Asymmetry, hollows in rounding contour, or winged scapula.

Palpate sternoclavicular and acromioclavicular joints, clavicle, scapulae, coracoid process, greater trochanter of humerus, biceps groove, area muscles

Palpate the biceps groove by rotating the arm and forearm externally. Follow the biceps muscle and tendon along the anterior aspect of the humerus into the biceps groove.

EXPECTED: No tenderness or masses, bilateral symmetry.

Palpate the muscle insertion for the supraspinatus, infraspinatus, and teres minor near the greater tuberosity of the humerus by lifting the elbow posteriorly to extend the shoulder.

UNEXPECTED: Pain, tenderness, mass.

Technique	Findings
Test range of motion Ask patient to perform the following movements:	
• *Shoulder shrug*	**EXPECTED:** Symmetric rising.
• *Forward flexion* Raise both arms forward and straight up over head.	**EXPECTED:** 180-degree forward flexion.
• *Hyperextension* Extend and stretch both arms behind back.	**EXPECTED:** 50-degree hyperextension.
• *Abduction* Lift both arms laterally and straight up over head.	**EXPECTED:** 180-degree abduction.
• *Adduction* Swing each arm across front of body.	**EXPECTED:** 50-degree adduction.
• *Internal rotation* Place both arms behind hips, elbows out.	**EXPECTED:** 90-degree internal rotation.
• *External rotation* Place both arms behind head, elbows out.	**EXPECTED:** 90-degree external rotation.
Test shoulder girdle muscle strength Ask patient to maintain the following positions while you apply opposing force:	
• *Shrugged shoulders* (This also tests cranial nerve XI.)	**EXPECTED:** Bilaterally symmetric with full resistance to opposition. **UNEXPECTED:** Inability to produce full resistance.

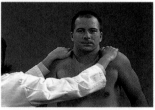

Shrugged shoulders.

• *Forward flexion*	**EXPECTED:** Bilaterally symmetric with full resistance to opposition. **UNEXPECTED:** Inability to produce full resistance.

Technique	Findings
• *Abduction*	**EXPECTED:** Bilaterally symmetric with full resistance to opposition. **UNEXPECTED:** Inability to produce full resistance.

Assess rotator cuff muscles

Technique	Findings
Abduct the arm 90 degrees and flex the shoulders forward 30 degrees to test the supraspinatus muscle. Apply downward pressure on the distal humerus when the arm is rotated so that thumb points down or up.	**UNEXPECTED:** Pain and weakness with opposing force.
Flex the elbow 90 degrees and rotate the forearm medially against resistance to test the subscapularis muscle.	**UNEXPECTED:** Pain and weakness with opposing force.
With the arm at the side and elbow flexed 90 degrees, rotate the arm laterally against resistance to test the infraspinatus and teres minor muscles.	**UNEXPECTED:** Pain and weakness with opposing force.

Evaluate the rotator cuff for impingement or a tear

Technique	Findings
• *Neer test:* Have the patient internally rotate and forward flex the arm at the shoulder, pressing the supraspinatus muscle against the anterior inferior acromion.	**UNEXPECTED:** Increased shoulder pain.
• *Hawkins test:* Abduct the shoulder to 90 degrees, flexing the elbow to 90 degrees, and then internally rotating the arm to its limit.	**UNEXPECTED:** Increased shoulder pain.

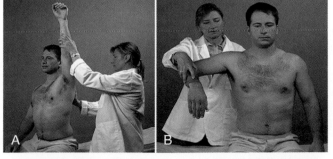

Assessment for rotator cuff inflammation or tear. **A,** Neer test. **B,** Hawkins test.

MUSCULOSKELETAL SYSTEM

Technique	Findings

Temporomandibular Joint

Palpate joint space for clicking, popping, pain

Locate temporomandibular joints with fingertips placed just anterior to tragus of each ear, as shown in figure at right. Ask patient to open mouth and allow fingertips to slip into joint space. Gently palpate.

EXPECTED: Audible or palpable snapping or clicking may be noted.
UNEXPECTED: Pain, crepitus, locking, or popping.

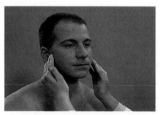

Palpating temporomandibular joint.

Test range of motion
Ask patient to:

• *Open and close mouth*

EXPECTED: Opens 3–6 cm between upper and lower teeth.

• *Move jaw laterally to each side*

EXPECTED: Mandible moves 1–2 cm in each direction.

• *Protrude and retract jaw*

EXPECTED: Both protrusion and retraction possible.

Test strength of temporalis and masseter muscles with patient's teeth clenched

Ask patient to clench teeth while you palpate contracted muscles and apply opposing force. (This also tests cranial nerve V motor function.)

EXPECTED: Bilaterally symmetric with full resistance to opposition.
UNEXPECTED: Inability to produce full resistance.

Cervical Spine

Inspect neck from anterior and posterior positions

• *Alignment*

EXPECTED: Cervical spine straight, with head erect and in approximate alignment.

• *Symmetry of skinfolds*

UNEXPECTED: Asymmetric skinfolds, webbed neck.

Technique	Findings
Palpate posterior neck, cervical spine, and paravertebral, trapezius, and sternocleidomastoid muscles	
	EXPECTED: Good muscle tone, symmetry in size. UNEXPECTED: Palpable tenderness or muscle spasm.
Test range of motion	
• *Forward flexion* Bend head forward, chin to chest.	EXPECTED: 45-degree flexion.
• *Hyperextension* Bend head backward, chin toward ceiling.	EXPECTED: 45-degree hyperextension.
• *Lateral bending* Bend head to each side, ear to each shoulder.	EXPECTED: 40-degree lateral bending.
• *Rotation* Turn head to each side, chin to shoulder.	EXPECTED: 70-degree rotation.
Test strength of sternocleidomastoid and trapezius muscles	
Ask patient to maintain each of the previous positions while you apply opposing force. (Cranial nerve XI is also tested with rotation.)	EXPECTED: Bilaterally symmetric strength with full resistance to opposition. UNEXPECTED: Inability to produce full resistance.

Thoracic and Lumbar Spine

Inspect spine for alignment

Note major landmarks of back—each spinal process of vertebrae (C7 and T1 usually most prominent), scapulae, iliac crests, paravertebral muscles.	EXPECTED: Head positioned directly over gluteal cleft, vertebrae straight (as indicated by symmetric shoulder, scapular, and iliac crest heights), curves of cervical and lumbar spines concave, curve of thoracic spine convex, and knees and feet aligned with trunk and pointing directly forward. UNEXPECTED: Lordosis, kyphosis, scoliosis, or sharp angular deformity (gibbus).

MUSCULOSKELETAL SYSTEM

Technique	Findings
Palpate spinal processes and paravertebral muscles Ask patient to stand erect.	**UNEXPECTED:** Muscle spasm or spinal tenderness.
Percuss for spinal tenderness Patient is still standing erect. First, tap each spinal process with one finger, then rap each side of spine along paravertebral muscles with ulnar aspect of fist.	**UNEXPECTED:** Muscle spasm or spinal tenderness.
Test range of motion and curvature Ask patient to perform the following movements (mark each spinal process with skin pencil if unexpected curvature suspected):	
• *Forward flexion* Bend forward at waist and try to touch toes. Observe patient from behind to check curvature.	**EXPECTED:** 75- to 90-degree flexion; back remains symmetrically flat as concave curve of lumbar spine becomes convex with forward flexion. **UNEXPECTED:** Lateral curvature or rib hump.
• *Hyperextension* Bend back at waist as far as possible.	**EXPECTED:** 30-degree hyperextension with reversal of lumbar curve.
• *Lateral bending* Bend to each side as far as possible.	**EXPECTED:** 35-degree lateral bending on each side.
• *Rotation* Swing upper trunk from waist in circular motion, front to side to back to side, while you stabilize pelvis.	**EXPECTED:** 30-degree rotation forward and backward.
Test for lumbar nerve root irritation or disk herniation at L4, L5, or S1 levels (patient supine with neck slightly flexed)	
• *Straight-leg raising test* Ask patient to raise leg with knee extended. Repeat with other leg.	**EXPECTED:** No pain below knee with leg raising. **UNEXPECTED:** Unable to raise leg more than 30 degrees without pain. Pain below knee in dermatome pattern. Flexion of knee often eliminates pain with leg raising. Crossover pain in affected leg.

Technique	Findings
• *Bragard stretch test* Hold patient's lower leg with knee extended, and raise it slowly until pain is felt. Lower leg slightly, briskly dorsiflex foot, and internally rotate hip.	**UNEXPECTED:** Pain when leg is raised less than 70 degrees; aggravated by dorsiflexion and internal rotation of hip.

Hips

Inspect hips for symmetry and level of gluteal folds

With patient standing, inspect anteriorly and posteriorly, using major landmarks of iliac crest and greater trochanter of femur.	**UNEXPECTED:** Asymmetry in iliac crest height, size of buttocks, or number and level of gluteal folds.

Test range of motion

While in position indicated, patient should perform the following movements:

• *Flexion, knee extended* With patient supine, raise leg over body.	**EXPECTED:** Up to 90-degree flexion.
• *Hyperextension* While standing or prone, swing straightened leg behind body without arching the back.	**EXPECTED:** Up to 30-degree hyperextension.
• *Flexion, knee flexed* While supine, raise one knee to chest while keeping other leg straight.	**EXPECTED:** 120-degree flexion.
• *Abduction and adduction* While supine, swing leg laterally and medially with knee straight. During adduction movement, lift patient's opposite leg to permit examined leg full movement.	**EXPECTED:** Some degree of both abduction and adduction.
• *Internal rotation* While supine, flex knee and rotate leg inward toward other leg.	**EXPECTED:** 40-degree internal rotation.
• *External rotation* While supine, place lateral aspect of foot on knee of other leg. Move flexed leg toward table.	**EXPECTED:** 45-degree external rotation.

Technique	Findings
Test hip muscle strength	
• *Knee in flexion and extension* Ask patient to maintain flexion of hip with knee in flexion and then extension while applying opposing force.	**EXPECTED:** Bilaterally symmetric with full resistance to opposition.
• *Resistance to uncrossing legs while seated*	**UNEXPECTED:** Inability to produce full resistance. **EXPECTED:** Bilaterally symmetric with full resistance to opposition.

Perform Trendelenburg test to inspect for weak hip abductor muscles

Ask patient to stand and balance first on one foot, then on other. Observe from behind.

UNEXPECTED: Asymmetry or change in level of iliac crests.

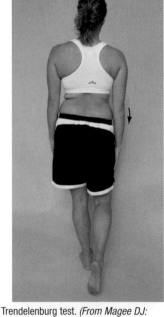

Trendelenburg test. *(From Magee DJ: Orthopedic physical assessment, ed 5, St Louis, 2007, Saunders.)*

Technique	Findings

Legs and Knees

Inspect knees and popliteal spaces, flexed and extended

Note major landmarks—tibial tuberosity, medial and lateral tibial condyles, medial and lateral epicondyles of femur, adductor tubercle of femur, patella.

EXPECTED: Natural concavities on anterior aspect, on each side, above patella.
UNEXPECTED: Convex rather than usual concave indentation above patella.

Observe lower leg alignment

EXPECTED: Angle between femur and tibia less than 15 degrees. Bowlegs common until 18 months of age; knock-knees common between 2 and 4 years.
UNEXPECTED: Knock-knees (genu valgum) or bowlegs (genu varum) at other ages, excessive hyperextension of knee with weight bearing (genu recurvatum).

Palpate popliteal space

UNEXPECTED: Swelling or tenderness.

Palpate tibiofemoral joint space
Identify patella, suprapatellar pouch, infrapatellar fat pad.

EXPECTED: Smooth and firm joint.
UNEXPECTED: Tenderness, bogginess, nodules, or crepitus.

Test range of motion
• *Flexion*
  Ask patient to bend each knee.

EXPECTED: 130-degree flexion.

• *Extension*
  Ask patient to straighten leg and stretch it.

EXPECTED: Full extension and up to 15-degree hyperextension.

Test muscle strength
• *Flexion and extension*
  Ask patient to maintain flexion and extension while you apply opposing force.

EXPECTED: Bilaterally symmetric with full resistance to opposition.
UNEXPECTED: Inability to produce full resistance.

Technique	Findings

Additional Techniques for Knees

Perform ballottement procedure to determine presence of excess fluid or effusion in knee

With knee extended, apply downward pressure on suprapatellar pouch with thumb and finger of one hand, then push patella sharply downward against femur with fingers of other hand, as shown in figure at right. Suddenly release pressure on patella, while keeping fingers lightly on knee.

UNEXPECTED: A tapping or clicking is sensed when patella is pushed against femur. Patella then floats out as if a fluid wave were pushing it.

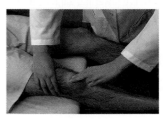

Ballottement.

Test for bulge sign to determine presence of excess fluid in knee

With knee extended, milk medial aspect of knee upward two or three times, as shown in figure below, *A*, then tap lateral side of patella, as shown below in figure, *B*.

UNEXPECTED: Bulge of returning fluid to hollow area medial to patella.

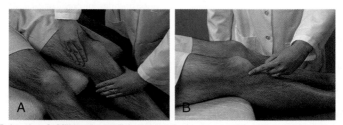

Bulge sign. **A,** Milking the medial aspect of the knee two or three times. **B,** Tap the lateral side of the patella.

Technique	Findings

Perform McMurray test to detect torn medial or lateral meniscus

Ask patient to lie supine and flex one knee completely with foot flat on table near buttocks. Maintain that flexion with your thumb and index finger on either side of the joint space while stabilizing knee. Hold heel with other hand; rotate foot and lower leg to lateral position. Extend knee to 90-degree angle. Return knee to full flexion, then repeat procedure rotating foot and lower leg to medial position.

UNEXPECTED: Palpable or audible click or limited extension of knee with either lateral or medial movements.

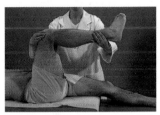

Procedure for examination of the knee with the McMurray test. Knee is flexed after lower leg was rotated to medial position.

Perform drawer test to identify instability of anterior and posterior cruciate ligaments

Ask patient, while supine, to flex knee 45–90 degrees, placing foot flat on table. Place both hands on lower leg with thumbs on ridge of anterior tibia near tibial tuberosity. Pull tibia, sliding it forward of femur. Then push tibia backward.

UNEXPECTED: Anterior or posterior movement greater than 5 mm.

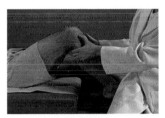

Drawer test.

Perform varus and valgus stress test to identify mediolateral collateral ligament instability

Ask patient to lie supine and extend knee. While you stabilize femur with one hand and hold ankle with other, apply varus force against the ankle (toward midline) and internal rotation.

UNEXPECTED: Excessive laxity felt as joint opening, medial or lateral movement.

Technique	Findings
Then apply valgus force against the ankle (away from midline) and external rotation. Repeat with knee flexed to 30 degrees.	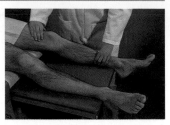

Varus and valgus stress test.

Feet and Ankles

Inspect during weight bearing (standing and walking) and non–weight bearing

Note major landmarks—medial malleolus, lateral malleolus, Achilles tendon.

- *Characteristics*

  EXPECTED: Smooth and rounded malleolar prominence, prominent heels, prominent metatarsophalangeal joints.
  UNEXPECTED: Calluses and corns.

- *Alignment*

  EXPECTED: Feet aligned with tibias and weight bearing on foot midline.
  UNEXPECTED: In-toeing (pes varus), out-toeing (pes valgus), deviations in forefoot alignment (metatarsus varus or metatarsus valgus), heel pronation, or pain.

- *Contour*

  EXPECTED: Longitudinal arch that may flatten with weight bearing. Foot flat when not bearing weight (pes planus) and high instep (pes cavus) are common variations.
  UNEXPECTED: Pain with pes planus.

- *Toes*

  EXPECTED: Toes on each foot straight forward, flat, in alignment.
  UNEXPECTED: Hammertoe; claw toe; mallet toe; hallux valgus; bunions; or heat, redness, swelling, tenderness of metatarsophalangeal joint of great toe (possibly with draining tophus).

Technique	Findings

Palpate Achilles tendon and each metatarsal joint

Using thumb and fingers of both hands, compress forefoot, palpating each metatarsophalangeal joint.

EXPECTED: No tenderness or masses, bilateral symmetry.
UNEXPECTED: Pain, masses, thickened Achilles tendon.

Test range of motion

Ask patient to sit, then perform following movements:

* *Dorsiflexion*
  Point foot toward ceiling.

EXPECTED: 20-degree dorsiflexion.

* *Plantar flexion*
  Point foot toward floor.

EXPECTED: 15-degree plantar flexion.

* *Inversion and eversion*
  Bend foot at ankle, then turn sole of foot toward and away from other foot.

EXPECTED: 30-degree inversion and 20-degree eversion.

* *Abduction and adduction*
  Rotate ankle, turning away from and then toward other foot (while you stabilize leg).

EXPECTED: 10-degree abduction and 20-degree adduction.

* *Flexion and extension*
  Bend and straighten toes.

EXPECTED: Some flexion and extension, especially of great toes.

Test strength of ankle muscles

Ask patient to maintain dorsiflexion and plantar flexion while you apply opposing force.

EXPECTED: Bilaterally symmetric with full resistance to opposition.
UNEXPECTED: Inability to produce full resistance.

AIDS TO DIFFERENTIAL DIAGNOSIS

Subjective Data	Objective Data

Ankylosing Spondylitis

Develops predominantly in male individuals between 20 and 40 years of age. Begins insidiously with low back pain, also involving hips and shoulders. Pain can fluctuate from one side to the other and progress to reduced spinal mobility.

Restriction in the lumbar flexion of the patient. The shoulders, hips, and knees may be affected later, developing limited range of motion. Uveitis may be present.

Subjective Data	Objective Data

Carpal Tunnel Syndrome

Numbness, burning, and tingling in the hands often occur at night. Can also be elicited by rotational movements of the wrist. Pain may radiate to the arms.

Weakness of the hand and flattening of the thenar eminence of the palm may result.

Gout

Sudden onset of a hot, swollen joint; exquisite pain; limited range of motion. Primarily affects men older than 40 years and women of postmenopausal age. Classically affects the proximal phalanx of the great toe, although the wrists, hands, ankles, and knees may be involved.

The skin over the swollen joint may be shiny and red or purple. Uric acid crystals may form as tophi under the skin with chronic gout.

Lumbar Disk Herniation

Can be associated with lifting heavy objects. Common symptoms include low back pain with radiation to the buttocks and posterior thigh or down the leg in the distribution of the dermatome of the nerve root. Pain relief is often achieved by lying down.

Spasm and tenderness over the paraspinal musculature may also be present. Patient may have difficulty with heel walking (L4 and L5) or toe walking (S1). Numbness, tingling, or weakness may occur in the involved extremity.

Bursitis

Common sites include the shoulder, elbow, hip, and knee with pain and stiffness surrounding the joint around the inflamed bursa. The pain usually is worse during activity.

Limitation of motion caused by swelling; pain on movement; point tenderness; and an erythematous, warm site. Soreness may radiate to tendons at the site.

Osteoarthritis

See table on p. ◆◆◆.

Rheumatoid Arthritis

See table on p. ◆◆◆.

MUSCULOSKELETAL SYSTEM

Subjective Data	Objective Data
Sprain Often associated with improper exercise warm-up, fatigue, or previous injury. Severity ranges from a mild intrafibrinous tear to a total rupture of a single muscle.	Temporary muscle weakness, spasm, pain, and contusion.
Fracture Usually occurs in the setting of acute trauma. Can occur more easily in patients with bone disorders (e.g., osteogenesis imperfecta, osteoporosis, bone metastasis).	Deformity, edema, pain, loss of function, color changes, and paresthesia.
Tenosynovitis (tendinitis) Pain with movement of such common sites as the shoulder, knee, heel, and wrist.	Point tenderness over the involved tendon. Pain with active movement, and some limitation of movement in the affected joint.
Rotator Cuff Tear May be pain in the shoulder and deltoid area that can awaken the patient at night.	May be an inability to maintain a lateral raised arm against resistance. Tenderness over the acromioclavicular joint. Grating sound on movement, crepitus, and weakness in external shoulder rotation.

Differential Diagnosis of Arthritis

Signs and Symptoms	Osteoarthritis	Rheumatoid Arthritis
Onset	Insidious	Gradual or sudden (24–48 hours)
Duration of stiffness	Few minutes, localized, but short "gelling" after prolonged rest	Often hours, most pronounced after rest
Pain	On motion, with prolonged activity, relieved by rest	Even at rest, may disturb sleep
Weakness	Usually localized and not severe	Often pronounced, out of proportion with muscle atrophy

Continued

MUSCULOSKELETAL SYSTEM

Differential Diagnosis of Arthritis—cont'd

Signs and Symptoms	Osteoarthritis	Rheumatoid Arthritis
Fatigue	Unusual	Often severe, with onset 4–5 hours after rising
Emotional depression and lability	Unusual	Common, coincides with fatigue and disease activity, often relieved if in remission
Tenderness over localized afflicted joint	Common	Almost always; most sensitive indicator of inflammation
Swelling	Effusion common, little synovial, reaction swelling rare	Fusiform soft tissue enlargement, effusion common, synovial proliferation and thickening
Heat, erythema	Unusual	Sometimes present
Crepitus, crackling	Coarse to medium on motion	Medium to fine
Joint enlargement	Mild with firm consistency	Moderate to severe

PEDIATRIC VARIATIONS

EXAMINATION

Musculoskeletal findings and motor development in infants, children, and adolescents change as they grow. (For a complete description of age-specific anticipated pediatric findings, see Chapter 21.)

Sports Participation Screening Examination for Children and Adolescents

- Observe posture and general muscle contour bilaterally.
- Observe gait.
- Ask patient to walk on tiptoes and heels.
- Observe patient hop on each foot.
- Ask patient to duck-walk four steps with knees completely bent.
- Inspect spine for curvature and lumbar extension, fingers touching toes with knees straight.
- Palpate shoulder and clavicle for dislocation.
- Check the following for range of motion—neck, shoulder, elbow, forearm, hands, fingers, hips.
- Test knee ligaments for drawer sign.

SAMPLE DOCUMENTATION

Subjective. A 13-year-old girl referred by school nurse because of uneven shoulder and hip heights. Active in sports, good strength, no back pain or stiffness.

Objective. Spine straight without obvious deformities when erect, but mild right curvature of thoracic spine with forward flexion. No rib hump. Right shoulder and iliac crest slightly higher than left. Muscles and extremities symmetric; muscle strength appropriate and equal bilaterally; active range of motion without pain, locking, clicking, or limitation in all joints.

CHAPTER 19

Neurologic System

EQUIPMENT

- Penlight
- Familiar objects (coins, keys, paper clip)
- Sterile needles
- Cotton wisp
- Tongue blades (one intact and one broken with pointed and rounded edges)
- Cup of water
- Tuning forks, 200 to 400 Hz and 500 to 1000 Hz
- Reflex hammer
- 5.07 monofilament
- Test tubes of hot and cold water
- Vials of aromatic substances (coffee, orange, peppermint, banana)
- Vials of solutions (glucose, salt, lemon or vinegar, quinine) with applicators
- List of tastes

EXAMINATION

Assess the neurologic system as the rest of the body is examined. When history and examination findings have not revealed a potential neurologic problem, perform a neurologic screening examination as shown in the box on pp. 218-219, rather than a full neurologic examination. See Chapter 18 for evaluation of muscle tone and strength, because these findings are important for interpreting neurologic system examination findings. The mental status portion of the neurologic system examination can be found in Chapter 3.

Neurologic Screening Examination

This shorter screening examination is commonly used for health visits when no known neurologic problem is apparent.

Cranial Nerves
Cranial nerves (CNs) II through XII are routinely tested; however, taste and smell are not tested unless some aberration is found (pp. 220-224).

NEUROLOGIC SYSTEM

Neurologic Screening Examination—cont'd

Proprioception and Cerebellar Function
One test is administered for each of the following: rapid rhythmic alternating movements, accuracy of movements, balance (Romberg test), gait, and heel-toe walking (pp. 224-226).

Sensory Function
Superficial pain and touch at a distal point in each extremity are tested; vibration and position senses are assessed by testing the great toe (pp. 226-232).

Deep Tendon Reflexes
All deep tendon reflexes and the plantar reflex are tested, excluding the test for clonus (pp. 232-235).

CRANIAL NERVES I TO XII

The following table summarizes the CN examination, and details of examination follow on pp. 220-224. When a sensory or motor loss is suspected, be compulsive about determining the extent of the loss.

Procedures for Cranial Nerve Examination

Cranial Nerve (CN)	Procedure
CN I (olfactory)	Test ability to identify familiar aromatic odors, one naris at a time with eyes closed.
CN II (optic)	Test distance and near vision.
	Perform an ophthalmoscopic examination.
	Test visual fields by confrontation and extinction of vision.
CN III, CN IV, CN VI (oculomotor, trochlear, abducens)	Test extraocular movement.
	Inspect eyelids for drooping.
	Inspect pupil size for equality, and direct and consensual response to light and accommodation.
CN V (trigeminal)	Inspect face for muscle atrophy and tremors.
	Palpate jaw muscles for tone and strength when patient clenches teeth.
	Test superficial pain and touch sensation in each nerve branch.
	(Test temperature sensation if findings to pain and touch sensation are unexpected.)
	Test corneal reflex.

Continued

NEUROLOGIC SYSTEM

Procedures for Cranial Nerve Examination—cont'd

Cranial Nerve (CN)	Procedure
CN VII (facial)	Inspect symmetry of facial features with various expressions (e.g., smile, frown, puffed cheeks, wrinkled forehead).
	Test ability to identify sweet, salty, sour, and bitter tastes on each side of tongue.
CN VIII (acoustic)	Test sense of hearing with whisper screening tests or by audiometry.
	Compare bone and air conduction of sound.
	Test for lateralization of sound.
CN IX (glossopharyngeal)	Test taste sensation (see CN VII).
	Test gag reflex and ability to swallow.
CN X (vagus)	Inspect palate and uvula for symmetry with speech sounds and gag reflex.
	Observe for swallowing difficulty.
	Evaluate quality of guttural speech sounds (presence of nasal or hoarse quality to voice).
CN XI (spinal accessory)	Test trapezius muscle strength (shrug shoulders against resistance).
	Test sternocleidomastoid muscle strength (turn head to each side against resistance).
CN XII (hypoglossal)	Inspect tongue in mouth and while protruded for symmetry, tremors, atrophy.
	Inspect tongue movement toward nose and chin.
	Test tongue strength with index finger when tongue is pressed against cheek.
	Evaluate quality of lingual speech sounds (*l, t, d, n*).

Technique	Findings
Assess olfactory nerve (CN I)	
Ask patient to close eyes. Occlude one naris, hold vial (using least irritating aromatic substances first [e.g., orange or peppermint extract]) under nose, and ask patient to breathe deeply and identify odor. Allow patient to breathe comfortably, then occlude other naris and repeat with different odor. Continue, alternating two or three odors.	**EXPECTED:** Able to perceive and usually identify odor on each side. **UNEXPECTED:** Anosmia, loss of smell or inability to discriminate odors.

NEUROLOGIC SYSTEM

Technique	Findings

Assess optic nerve (CN II)
See tests for near and distance visual acuity and visual fields in Chapter 8.

EXPECTED: Vision 20/20 without or with lenses each eye; full visual fields.

Assess oculomotor, trochlear, abducens nerves (CN III, CN IV, CN VI)
See tests for six cardinal points of gaze, pupil size, shape, response to light and accommodation, and opening of upper eyelids in Chapter 8.

EXPECTED: Equal pupil size, equal and consensual response to light and accommodation, symmetric eye movements in all six cardinal points of gaze.
UNEXPECTED: Absence of lateral gaze. Absence of any expected finding, ptosis.

Assess trigeminal nerve (CN V)
* *Facial muscle tone*
  Inspect face for symmetry or muscle twitching. Ask patient to clench teeth tightly as you palpate muscles over jaw.

EXPECTED: Symmetric tone.
UNEXPECTED: Muscle atrophy, deviation of jaw to one side, or fasciculations.

* *Sensation*
  Ask patient to close eyes and report if sensation to touch is sharp or dull as you touch each side of face at scalp, cheek, and chin areas, alternately using sharp and rounded edges of tongue blade or paper clip in an unpredictable pattern. Ask patient to report when the stimulus is felt as you stroke same six areas with cotton wisp or brush. Finally, test sensation over buccal mucosa with wooden applicator.

EXPECTED: Symmetric discrimination of sensations in each location to all stimuli.
UNEXPECTED: Impaired sensation with identified distribution. If impaired, use test tubes of hot and cold water to evaluate temperature sensation.

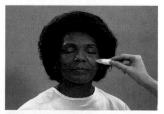

Testing sensation over distribution of cranial nerve V.

* *Corneal reflex*
  See test for corneal sensitivity in Chapter 8.

EXPECTED: Symmetric blink reflex. May be diminished or absent if patient wears contact lenses.

Technique	Findings

Assess facial nerve (CN VII)

* *Expressions*

  Assess motor function by asking patient to make the following facial expressions:
  + Raise eyebrows and wrinkle forehead
  + Smile
  + Frown
  + Puff out cheeks
  + Purse lips and blow out
  + Show teeth
  + Squeeze eyes shut against resistance

EXPECTED: Facial symmetry.
UNEXPECTED: Tics, unusual facial movements, or asymmetry of expression (flattened nasolabial fold, lower eyelid sagging, side of mouth drooping).

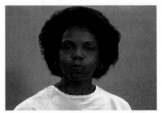

Assessing motor function of cranial nerve VII.

* *Speech*

  Listen to articulation and clarity of speech

UNEXPECTED: Difficulty with enunciation of *b*, *m*, and *p* (labial sounds).

* *Taste (CN VII and CN IX)*

  Hold card listing tastes in patient's view. Ask patient to extend tongue. Apply one of four solutions to lateral side of tongue in appropriate taste-bud region. Ask patient to point to taste perceived. Offer patient a sip of water, and repeat with different solution and applicator, testing each side of tongue with each solution.

EXPECTED: Able to identify sweet, salty, sour, bitter taste bilaterally when placed in appropriate taste-bud region.

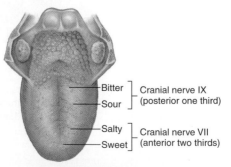

Sites for taste assessment.

Technique	Findings
Assess acoustic nerve (CN VIII)	
• *Hearing* See screening tests in Chapter 9 or use an audiometer to test hearing.	**EXPECTED:** Adequate hearing bilaterally.
• *Balance* See Romberg test on p. 225.	
Assess glossopharyngeal nerve (CN IX)	
• *Taste* See CN VII.	
• *Gag reflex (nasopharyngeal sensation)* See CN X.	
Assess vagus nerve (CN X)	
• *Motor function* Ask patient to say "aah" while observing movement of palate and uvula.	**EXPECTED:** Soft palate rises with uvula in midline. **UNEXPECTED:** Failure of soft palate to rise or uvula deviates from midline.
• *Gag reflex (nasopharyngeal sensation; CN IX and CN X)* Tell patient you will be testing gag reflex. Touch posterior wall of pharynx with applicator while observing palate, pharyngeal muscles, and uvula.	**EXPECTED:** Upward movement of palate and contraction of pharyngeal muscles, with uvula in midline. **UNEXPECTED:** Drooping or absence of arch on either side of soft palate; uvula deviates from midline.
• *Swallowing (CN IX and CN X)* Ask patient to swallow water.	**EXPECTED:** Water easily swallowed. **UNEXPECTED:** Retrograde passage of water through nose.
• *Speech*	**UNEXPECTED:** Hoarseness, nasal quality, or difficulty with guttural sounds.
Assess spinal accessory nerve (CN XI) See Chapters 7 and 18 for evaluations of size, shape, strength of trapezius and sternocleidomastoid muscles.	**EXPECTED:** Symmetric size, shape, and strength.

NEUROLOGIC SYSTEM

Technique	Findings

Assess hypoglossal nerve (CN XII)

- *Tongue resting and protruded*
  Inspect while at rest on floor of mouth and while protruded.

EXPECTED: Tongue midline, symmetric size.
UNEXPECTED: Fasciculations, asymmetry, atrophy, or deviation from midline.

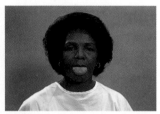

Assessing motor function of cranial nerve XII.

- *Tongue movement*
  Ask patient to move tongue in and out, side to side, curled up toward nose, curled down toward chin.

EXPECTED: Able to perform most tongue movements.

- *Tongue strength*
  Ask patient to push tongue against cheek while you apply resistance with index finger.

EXPECTED: Steady, firm pressure.

- *Speech*

UNEXPECTED: Problems with *l*, *t*, *d*, or *n* (lingual sounds).

Proprioception and Cerebellar Function
Evaluate coordination and fine motor skills

Have patient sit.
- *Rapid, rhythmic, alternating movements*
  Ask patient to pat knees with both hands, alternately patting with palmar and dorsal surfaces of the hands. Or ask the patient to touch the thumb to each finger of the same hand sequentially from index finger to little finger and back, one hand at a time.

EXPECTED: Smooth execution, maintaining rhythm with increasing speed.
UNEXPECTED: Stiff, slowed, nonrhythmic, or jerky clonic movements.

Technique	Findings
• *Accuracy of movement: Finger-to-nose test* Position your index finger 40–50 cm from patient. Ask patient to touch his or her nose and your index finger with the index finger of one hand, as shown below. Change location of your index finger several times. Repeat with patient's other hand. Alternatively ask the patient to close both eyes and touch his or her nose with index finger of each hand while alternating hands and gradually increasing speed.	**EXPECTED:** Movements rapid, smooth, accurate. **UNEXPECTED:** Consistent past pointing (missing examiner's index finger).

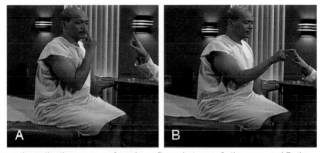

Assess the patient's accuracy of moving a finger between **A**, the nose, and **B**, the examiner's finger.

Technique	Findings
• *Accuracy of movement: Heel-to-shin test* (can be performed sitting, standing, or supine). Ask patient to run heel of one foot along shin of opposite leg from knee to ankle. Repeat with other heel.	**EXPECTED:** Able to move heel up and down shin in straight line. **UNEXPECTED:** Irregular deviations to side.

Evaluate balance

Technique	Findings
• *Balance: Romberg test* Ask patient to stand with feet together and arms at sides, with eyes first open, then closed. **Stand close by in case patient starts to fall.**	**EXPECTED:** Slight swaying movement, no danger of falling. **UNEXPECTED:** Staggering, losing balance, or swaying to the extent of falling.

NEUROLOGIC SYSTEM

Technique	Findings
• *Balance: Recovery* After explaining test to patient, ask patient to spread feet slightly, then push shoulders with enough effort to throw patient off balance. **Be prepared to catch patient.**	**EXPECTED:** Quick recovery of balance. **UNEXPECTED:** Must catch patient to prevent a fall.
• *Balance: Standing and hopping* Have patient (eyes closed) stand in place on one foot, then the other. Then have patient (with eyes open) hop on each foot.	**EXPECTED:** Able to stand and hop on each foot for 5 seconds without losing balance. **UNEXPECTED:** Instability, need to continually touch floor with opposite foot, or tendency to fall.
• *Gait: Walking* Ask patient to walk without shoes around examining room or down hallway, with eyes open, then closed.	**EXPECTED:** Smooth, regular gait rhythm and symmetric stride length; upright trunk posture swaying with gait phase; and arm swing smooth and symmetric. **UNEXPECTED:** Shuffling, widely placed feet, toe walking, foot flop, leg lag, scissoring, loss of arm swing, staggering, lurching, or waddling motion.
• *Gait: Heel-toe walking* Ask patient (arms at side and eyes open) to walk a straight line, first forward and then backward. Ask patient to touch toe of one foot with heel of other.	**EXPECTED:** Consistent contact between toe and heel, slight swaying. **UNEXPECTED:** Extension of arms for balance, instability, tendency to fall, or lateral staggering and reeling.

Sensory Function

Test primary sensory functions

Ask patient to close eyes for all tests. Use minimal stimulation initially, then increase gradually until patient becomes aware. Test contralateral areas, asking patient to compare perceived sensations side to side.	**EXPECTED:** For all tests, minimal differences side to side, correct interpretation of sensations (e.g., sharp, dull), distinguishes side of body tested and location of sensation (e.g., proximal or distal to previous stimulus). **UNEXPECTED:** For all tests, map boundaries of any impairment by distribution of major peripheral nerves or dermatomes (see figures on pp. 227-228).

Technique   Findings

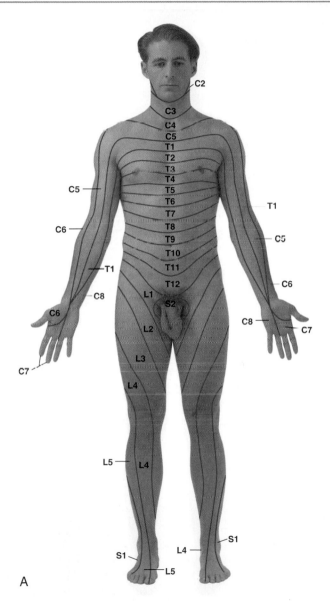

A

Technique	Findings

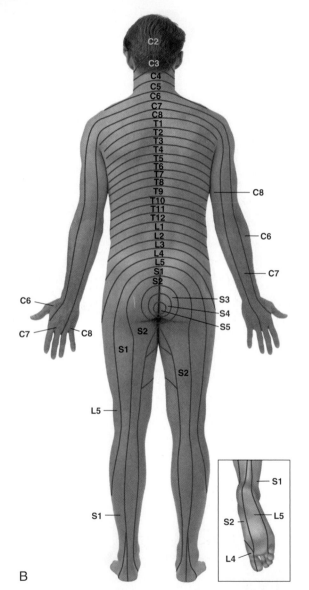

A, Dermatomes of the body, anterior view. **B,** Dermatomes of the body, posterior view.

Technique	Findings

- *Superficial touch*
  Lightly touch skin with cotton wisp or your fingertips, as shown at right. Ask patient to point to area touched or indicate when sensation is felt.

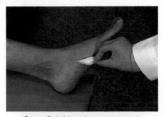

Superficial touch assessment.

- *Superficial pain*
  Alternate the sharp and smooth edges of broken tongue blade or round and end point of a paper clip, touching the skin in an unpredictable pattern. Allow 2 seconds between sensations. Ask patient to identify sensation (sharp or dull) and where it is felt.

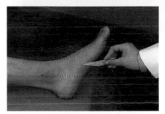

Superficial pain assessment.

- *Temperature and deep pressure*
  Perform test only if superficial pain sensation is not intact.
  - *Temperature:* Alternately roll test tubes of hot and cold water against skin in an unpredictable pattern. Ask patient to indicate hot or cold and where it is felt.

  EXPECTED: Distinguishes between hot and cold and location of sensation.

  - *Deep pressure:* Squeeze trapezius, calf, or biceps muscle.

  EXPECTED: Discomfort with deep pressure.

- *Protective sensation*
  Perform test only if patient has diabetes mellitus or impaired sensation is suspected.
  Apply 5.07 monofilament until filament bends. Use a random pattern to test several sites on plantar surface of foot and once on dorsal surface. Avoid calloused areas and broken skin.

  EXPECTED: Sensation felt at all sites touched.
  UNEXPECTED: Loss of sensation at any site.

NEUROLOGIC SYSTEM

Technique	Findings

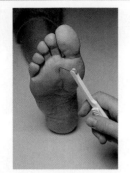

Monofilament testing of superficial touch.

- *Vibration*

  Place stem of vibrating tuning fork against several bony prominences (e.g., toes, ankle, shin, finger joints, wrist, elbow, shoulder, sternum), beginning distally. Ask patient when and where sensation is felt and what it feels like. Dampen tines occasionally to see whether patient notices the difference.

EXPECTED: Buzzing or tingling sensation, correct location of stimulus.

UNEXPECTED: Does not distinguish vibration from touch of nonvibrating tuning fork.

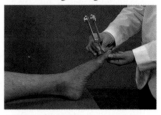

Assessment of vibration sensation.

- *Position of joints*

  Hold joint to be tested (great toe or finger) by lateral aspects in neutral position, then raise or lower the digit. Ask the patient which way the joint was moved. Return the digit to neutral before moving it another direction. Repeat and test a joint in both feet and both hands.

EXPECTED: Patient correctly identifies position of joint.

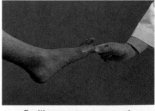

Position sense assessment.

Technique	Findings
Test cortical sensory functions	
Ask patient to close eyes for all tests.	
• *Stereognosis* Hand patient familiar objects (e.g., key, coin) and ask patient to identify by touch.	**UNEXPECTED:** Inability to recognize objects (tactile agnosia).

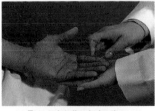

Stereognosis.

| • *Two-point discrimination*
 Use two sterile needles or two tongue blade sharp edges, to touch patient's skin with one or both points simultaneously at various locations. Find distance at which patient can no longer distinguish two points. | **EXPECTED:** Correctly identifies one or two point used. On the fingertips and toes, points are commonly felt when 2–8 mm apart. Discrimination of two points varies on other body parts, such as the back (40–70 mm) or chest and forearms (40 mm). |

Two-point discrimination.

| • *Extinction phenomenon*
 Use sharp points of a broken tongue blade to simultaneously touch cheek and hand, or two other areas on each side of body. Ask patient the number of stimuli and locations. | **EXPECTED:** Correct number and location of both sensations identified bilaterally. |

NEUROLOGIC SYSTEM

Technique	Findings
• *Graphesthesia* With blunt pen or applicator stick, draw letter, number, or shape on palm of patient's hand, and ask patient to identify it. Repeat with different figure on other hand.	**EXPECTED:** Letter, number, or figure readily recognized.

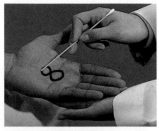

Graphesthesia.

• *Point location*
Touch area on patient's skin and withdraw stimulus. Ask patient to point to area touched.

EXPECTED: Able to locate stimulus.

Reflexes

Test superficial reflexes
Have patient supine.

• *Abdominal*
Stroke each quadrant of abdomen with end of reflex hammer or with tongue blade edge.

EXPECTED: Slight, bilaterally equal movement of umbilicus toward each area of stimulation. May have diminished response in obese patient or when abdominal muscles stretched by pregnancy.

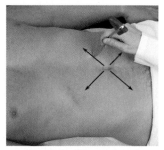

Abdominal reflex assessment.

• *Cremasteric (male patients)*
Stroke inner thigh, proximal to distal.

EXPECTED: Testicle and scrotum rise on stroked side.

NEUROLOGIC SYSTEM

Technique	Findings
• *Plantar reflex* Using pointed object, stroke lateral side of foot from heel to ball and then across ball of foot to medial side.	**EXPECTED:** Plantar flexion of all toes. Dorsiflexion of great toe and fanning of other toes in children younger than 2 years. **UNEXPECTED:** Fanning of toes or dorsiflexion of great toe with or without fanning of other toes (Babinski sign positive) in all patients older than 2 years.

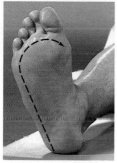

Plantar reflex assessment.

Test deep tendon reflexes

Patient relaxed and either sitting or lying for most procedures. Test each reflex, comparing responses side to side. Score deep tendon reflexes on scale shown in table below.	**EXPECTED:** Symmetric visible or palpable responses. **UNEXPECTED:** Absent or diminished responses (0 or 1+), or hyperactive reflexes (3+ or 4+).

Scoring Deep Tendon Reflexes

Grade	Deep Tendon Reflex Response
0	No response
1+	Sluggish or diminished
2+	Active or expected response
3+	More brisk than expected, slightly hyperactive
4+	Brisk, hyperactive, with intermittent or transient clonus

NEUROLOGIC SYSTEM

Technique	Findings

- *Biceps*
  Flex arm 45 degrees at elbow, then palpate biceps tendon in antecubital fossa. Place thumb over tendon and fingers under elbow. Strike your thumb with reflex hammer.

EXPECTED: Visible or palpable flexion of elbow, contraction of biceps muscle.

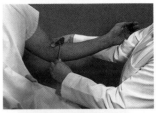

Biceps deep tendon reflex.

- *Brachioradial*
  Flex patient's arm up to 45 degrees while resting patient's forearm on your arm, with hand slightly pronated. Strike brachioradial tendon directly.

EXPECTED: Pronation of forearm and flexion of elbow.

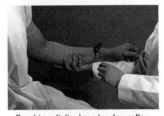

Brachioradialis deep tendon reflex.

- *Triceps*
  Flex patient's arm at elbow up to 90 degrees. Allow patient's lower arm to hang freely or rest patient's forearm on your arm. Palpate triceps tendon and strike directly with reflex hammer, just above elbow.

EXPECTED: Visible or palpable extension of elbow, contraction of triceps muscle.

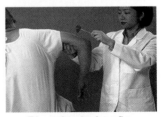

Triceps deep tendon reflex.

Technique	Findings

- *Patellar*
  Flex patient's knee up to 90 degrees, allowing lower leg to hang loosely. Support upper leg so it does not rest against edge of examining table, then strike patellar tendon just below patella.

EXPECTED: Extension of lower leg, contraction of quadriceps muscle.

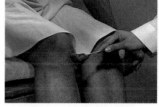

Patellar deep tendon reflex.

- *Achilles*
  Ask patient to sit. Then flex patient's knee and dorsiflex ankle up to 90 degrees, holding heel of foot. Strike Achilles tendon at level of ankle malleoli.

EXPECTED: Plantar flexion, contraction of gastrocnemius muscle.

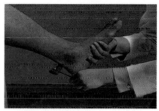

Achilles deep tendon reflex.

- *Clonus*
  Support patient's knee in partially flexed position and briskly dorsiflex foot with other hand, maintaining foot in flexion.

EXPECTED: No rhythmic oscillating movements.
UNEXPECTED: Sustained clonus, rhythmic oscillating movements between dorsiflexion and plantar flexion palpated.

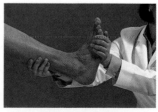

Clonus assessment.

Differential Diagnosis of Upper and Lower Motor Neuron Disorders

Assessment Parameters	Upper Motor Neuron	Lower Motor Neuron
Muscle tone	Increased tone, muscle spasticity, risk for contractures	Decreased tone, muscle flaccidity
Muscle atrophy	Little or no muscle atrophy, but decreased strength	Loss of muscle strength; muscle atrophy or wasting
Sensation	Sensation loss may affect entire limb	Sensory loss that follows the distribution of dermatomes or peripheral nerves
Reflexes	Hyperactive deep tendon and abdominal reflexes; positive Babinski sign	Weak or absent deep tendon, plantar, and abdominal reflexes, negative plantar reflex, no pathologic reflexes
Fasciculation	No fasciculations	Fasciculations
Motor effect	Paralysis of voluntary movements	Paralysis of muscles
Location of insult	Damage above level of brainstem will affect contralateral side of body, damage below the brainstem will affect the ipsilateral side of the body	Damage affects muscle on ipsilateral side of body

AIDS TO DIFFERENTIAL DIAGNOSIS

Subjective Data	Objective Data

Multiple Sclerosis

Fatigue; vertigo, weakness, numbness; blurred vision, diplopia, vision loss; urinary frequency, urgency, hesitancy; sexual dysfunction; emotional changes	Muscle weakness, ataxia; hyperactive deep tendon reflexes; paresthesias, sensory loss; intention tremor; optic neuritis; cognitive changes

Subjective Data	Objective Data

Generalized Seizure Disorder

Premonition or aura, stiff body followed by rhythmic jerking movements, eyes rolled upward, drooling; loss of bladder and bowel control

Tonic phase (brief flexion then extension for 10–15 minutes, eyes deviated upward, dilated pupils), clonic phase (alternating muscle contraction and relaxation), postictal (coma followed by confusion and lethargy)

Meningitis

Fever, chills, headache, stiff neck, lethargy, malaise, vomiting, irritability, seizures

Altered mental status, confusion, nuchal rigidity, may see positive Brudzinski and Kernig signs

Encephalitis

Recovery from mild viral illness with fever, then lethargy, restlessness, mental confusion

Altered mental status, confusion, stupor, coma, photophobia, stiff neck, muscle weakness, paralysis, ataxia

Intracranial Tumor

Headaches, may awaken from sleep; nausea and vomiting; memory loss and confusion; unsteady gait; impaired coordination; behavioral or personality changes

Signs vary by location of lesion; altered consciousness, confusion, papilledema, CN impairment, aphasia, vision loss, gait disturbance, ataxia

Stroke (cerebrovascular accident or brain attack)

Sudden numbness or weakness, often unilateral; sudden confusion, difficulty speaking or understanding speech; sudden trouble seeing in one or both eyes; sudden trouble walking, loss of balance, or loss of coordination; sudden severe headache with no known cause

Altered consciousness, elevated blood pressure, difficulty managing secretions, weakness or paralysis of extremities or facial muscles on one or both sides of body, aphasia (receptive or expressive), articulation impairment, impaired horizontal gaze or hemianopia

Parkinson Disease

Tremors at rest and with fatigue that disappear with intended movement and sleep; slowing of voluntary movement; bilateral pill rolling of fingers; may have numbness, aching, tingling and muscle soreness

Tremors; muscle rigidity; stooped posture; instability of balance; short steps, shuffling, freezing gait; difficulty swallowing, drooling, voice softening, slowed, slurred, monotonous speech; impaired cognition, dementia

NEUROLOGIC SYSTEM

Subjective Data	Objective Data
Peripheral Neuropathy Gradual onset of numbness, tingling, burning in hands and feet; sensation of walking on cotton or floors feel strange; inability of fingers to feel difference between coins; night pain in feet	Reduced protective sensation in foot and may progress up lower leg; distal pulses diminished, diminished ankle and knee deep tendon reflexes, loss of vibratory sensation below knee, distal muscle weakness, cannot stand on toes or heels
Trigeminal Neuralgia Sharp pain episodes on one side of face potentially caused by chewing, swallowing, talking, brushing teeth, or cold exposure	May have slight sensory impairment in regions of pain, may have normal neurologic findings
Bell's Palsy Rapidly progression of muscle weakness on one side of face, feeling of facial numbness	Facial creases and nasolabial fold disappear on affected side, eyelid does not close and lower lid sags on affected side, facial sensation is intact
Cerebral Palsy Delays in gross motor development, activity limitation; may have hearing, speech, or language disorders, feeding difficulties	Increased or decreased muscle tone, tremors, scissor gait or wide-based gait, toe walking, exaggerated posturing, mental retardation or learning disabilities, persistent primitive reflexes, inconsistent muscle tone

PEDIATRIC VARIATIONS

EXAMINATION

Neurologic findings in the infant and child change as the child matures. (For a complete description of expected developmental findings by age, see Chapter 21.)

Technique	Findings

Indirectly evaluate CNs in newborns and infants

- *Optical blink reflex (CN II, CN III, CN IV, CN VI)*
  Shine a light at infant's open eyes. Observe quick closure of eyes and dorsal flexion of head.

  EXPECTED: Gazes intensely at close object or face. Focuses on and tracks an object with both eyes.
  UNEXPECTED: No response may indicate poor light perception.

- *Rooting reflex (CN V)*
  Touch one corner of infant's mouth.

  EXPECTED: Infant should open mouth and turn head in direction of stimulation. If infant has been fed recently, minimal or no response is expected.

- *Sucking reflex (CN V)*
  Place your finger in infant's mouth, feeling sucking action. Note pressure, strength, pattern of sucking.

  EXPECTED: Tongue should push up against your finger with good strength.

- *Infant's facial expression (CN VII)*
  Note wrinkling of forehead when crying and symmetry of smile.

  EXPECTED: Facial symmetry with all expressions.

- *Acoustic blink reflex (CN VIII)*
  Loudly clap your hands about 30 cm from infant's head; avoid producing an air current.

  EXPECTED: Blink and movement of eyes in response to sound. Infant will habituate to repeated testing. Freezes position with high-pitched sound.
  UNEXPECTED: No response after 2–3 days of age.

- *Doll's eye maneuver (CN VIII)*
  Hold infant under axilla in upright position, head held steady, facing you. Rotate infant first in one direction and then in other.

  EXPECTED: Infant's eyes turn in direction of rotation and then opposite direction when rotation stops.
  UNEXPECTED: Eyes do not move in expected direction.

- *Swallowing and gag reflex (CN IX and CN X)*

  EXPECTED: Coordinated sucking and swallowing ability.

NEUROLOGIC SYSTEM

Technique	Findings
• *Sucking and swallowing (CN XII)* Pinch infant's nose.	EXPECTED: Mouth will open, and tip of tongue will rise in midline position.
Evaluate primitive reflexes in infant	
• *Palmar grasp (present at birth)* Making sure infant's head is in midline, touch palm of infant's hand from ulnar side (opposite thumb)	EXPECTED: Strong grasp of your finger. Sucking facilitates grasp. Grasp should be strongest between 1 and 2 months of age and disappear by 3 months.
• *Plantar grasp (present at birth)* Touch plantar surface of infant's feet at the base of toes.	EXPECTED: Toes should curl downward. Reflex should be strong up to 8 months of age.
• *Moro reflex (present at birth)* With infant supported in semisitting position, allow head and trunk to drop back to a 30-degree angle.	EXPECTED: Symmetric abduction and extension of arms. Fingers fan out, and thumb and index finger form a C. Arms then adduct in an embracing motion followed by relaxed flexion. Reflex diminishes in strength by 3–4 months and disappears by 6 months.
• *Placing (4 days of age)* Hold infant upright under axilla next to a table or chair. Touch dorsal side of foot to table or chair edge.	EXPECTED: Flexion of hip and knee, lifting of foot as if stepping up on table. Age of disappearance varies.
• *Stepping (between birth and 8 weeks)* Hold infant upright under axilla and allow soles of feet to touch surface of table.	EXPECTED: Alternate flexion and extension of legs, simulating walking. Disappears before voluntary walking.
• *Asymmetric tonic neck or "fencing" (by 2–3 months)* With infant lying supine and relaxed or sleeping, turn infant's head to one side so jaw is over shoulder. Then turn infant's head to other side.	EXPECTED: Extension of arm and leg on side to which head is turned and flexion of opposite arm and leg. Reversal of extremities' positions with head turned opposite way. Reflex diminishes by 3–4 months of age and disappears by 6 months. UNEXPECTED: Be concerned if infant never exhibits reflex or seems locked in fencing position.

SAMPLE DOCUMENTATION

Subjective. A 48-year-old man presents for his annual physical examination. No concerns about poor balance, loss of sensation, unsteady gait. History of diabetes mellitus type 1 for 30 years, well controlled.

Objective. CNs II to XII grossly intact. Gait is coordinated and even. Romberg negative. Rapid alternating movements coordinated and smooth. Superficial touch, pain, vibratory sensation are intact bilaterally. Deep tendon reflexes 2+ bilaterally in all extremities. Plantar reflex produces expected plantar flexion of toes. No ankle clonus. Monofilament test reveals decreased sensation on plantar surfaces of both feet.

NEUROLOGIC SYSTEM

CHAPTER 20

Head-to-Toe Examination: Adult

COMPONENTS OF THE EXAMINATION

There is no one correct way to order the parts of the physical examination. You are encouraged to consider and then to adapt and edit the following suggested approach for the unique needs of the particular patient and the relevant demands of the moment.

GENERAL INSPECTION

Start examination the moment the patient is within your view. As you first observe the patient, for example, in the waiting room, take note of the following characteristics:

- Signs of distress or disease
- Habitus
- Manner of sitting
- Degree of facial relaxation

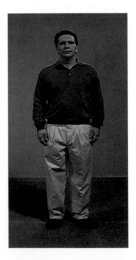

- Relationship with others in room
- Degree of interest in what is happening in room
- Manner with which you are met
- Moistness of palm when you shake hands
- Eyes—luster and expression of emotion
- Skin color
- Facial expression
- Mobility:
  - Use of assistive devices
  - Gait
  - Sitting, rising from chair
  - Taking off coat
  - Dress and posture
- Speech pattern, disorders, foreign language
- Difficulty hearing, assistive devices
- Stature and build
- Musculoskeletal deformities
- Vision problems, assistive devices
- Eye contact with you
- Orientation, mental alertness
- Nutritional state
- Respiratory problems
- Significant others accompanying patient

PATIENT INSTRUCTIONS (PLAN EACH STEP TO MINIMIZE THE PATIENT'S EFFORT AND TO CONSERVE ENERGY)

- Empty bladder.
- Remove as much clothing as is necessary (always respecting modesty).
- Put on a gown.

MEASUREMENTS

- Measure weight and calculate the body mass index.
- Measure height.
- Assess distance vision—Snellen chart.
- Document vital signs—temperature, pulse, respiration, blood pressure in both arms, pain assessment.

PATIENT SEATED, WEARING GOWN

Stand in front of patient seated on examining table.

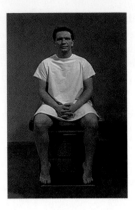

Head and Face

- Inspect skin characteristics.
- Inspect symmetry and external characteristics of eyes and ears.
- Inspect configuration of skull.
- Inspect and palpate scalp and hair for texture, distribution, and quantity of hair.
- Palpate facial bones.
- Palpate temporomandibular joint while patient opens and closes mouth.
- Palpate sinus regions; if tender, transilluminate them (may be helpful, but sensitivity and specificity are uncertain when considered separate from other findings).
- Inspect ability to clench teeth, squeeze eyes tightly shut, wrinkle forehead, smile, stick out tongue, and puff out cheeks (CN V, VII).
- Test sensation using light touch on forehead, cheeks, chin (CN V).

Eyes

- External examination:
  - Inspect eyelids, eyelashes, palpebral folds.
  - Determine alignment of eyebrows.
  - Inspect sclerae, conjunctivae, irides.
  - Palpate lacrimal apparatus.
  - Test near-vision—Rosenbaum chart (CN II).
- Eye function:
  - Test pupillary response to light and accommodation.
  - Perform cover-uncover test and corneal light reflex.
  - Test extraocular eye movements (CN III, IV, VI).
  - Assess visual fields (CN II).
  - Test corneal reflexes (CN V).

- Ophthalmoscopic examination:
  - Test red reflex.
  - Inspect lens.
  - Inspect disc, cup margins, vessels, retinal surface.

Ears
- Inspect alignment and placement.
- Inspect surface characteristics.
- Palpate auricle.
- Assess hearing with whisper test or ticking watch (CN VIII).
- Perform otoscopic examination:
  - Inspect canals.
  - Inspect tympanic membranes for landmarks, deformities, inflammation.
- Perform Rinne and Weber tests.

Nose
- Note structure, position of septum.
- Determine patency of each nostril.
- Inspect mucosa, septum, turbinates with nasal speculum.
- Assess sense of smell when clinically necessary (CN I).

Mouth and Pharynx
- Inspect lips, buccal mucosa, gums, hard and soft palates, floor of mouth for color and surface characteristics.
- Inspect oropharynx: note anteroposterior pillars, uvula, tonsils, posterior pharynx, mouth odor.
- Inspect teeth for color, number, surface characteristics.
- Inspect tongue for color, characteristics, symmetry, movement (CN XII).
- Test gag reflex and "ah" reflex (CN IX, X).
- Assess sense of taste test when clinically indicated (CN VII, IX).

Neck
- Inspect for symmetry and smoothness of neck and thyroid.
- Inspect for jugular venous distention (also when patient is supine).
- Perform active and passive range of motion; test resistance against examiner's hand.
- Test strength of shoulder shrug (CN IX).
- Palpate carotid pulses. Be sure to palpate one side at a time (also when patient is supine).
- Palpate tracheal position.
- Palpate thyroid.
- Palpate lymph nodes—preauricular and postauricular, occipital, tonsillar, submental, submandibular, superficial cervical chain, posterior cervical, deep cervical, supraclavicular.
- Auscultate carotid arteries and thyroid.

Upper Extremities

- Inspect skin and nail characteristics.
- Inspect symmetry of muscle mass.
- Inspect and palpate hands, arms, shoulders, including epitrochlear nodes; note musculoskeletal deformities.
- Assess joint range-of-motion and muscle strength: fingers, wrists, elbows, and shoulders.
- Assess pulses—radial, brachial.

PATIENT SEATED, BACK EXPOSED

Stand behind patient seated on examining table. Have male patients pull gown down to the waist so entire chest and back are exposed. Have females expose back; keep breasts covered.

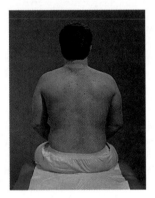

Back and Posterior Chest

- Inspect skin and thoracic configuration.
- Inspect symmetry of shoulders, musculoskeletal development.
- Inspect and palpate scapulae and spine.
- Palpate and percuss costovertebral angle.

Lungs

- Inspect respiration—excursion, depth, rhythm, pattern.
- Palpate for expansion and tactile fremitus.
- Palpate scapular and subscapular nodes.
- Percuss posterior chest and lateral walls systematically for resonance.
- Percuss for diaphragmatic excursion.
- Auscultate systematically for breath sounds. Note characteristics and adventitious sounds.

PATIENT SEATED, CHEST EXPOSED

Move around to front of patient. Have female patients lower gown to expose anterior chest.

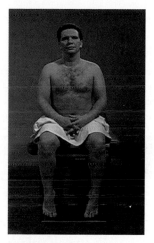

Anterior Chest, Lungs, Heart

- Inspect skin, musculoskeletal development, symmetry.
- Inspect respirations—patient posture, respiratory effort.
- Inspect for pulsations or heaving.
- Palpate chest wall for stability, crepitation, tenderness.
- Palpate precordium for thrills, heaves, pulsations, and location of apical impulse.
- Palpate for tactile fremitus.
- Palpate axillary nodes.
- Percuss systematically for resonance.
- Auscultate systematically for breath sounds.
- Auscultate systematically for heart sounds—aortic, pulmonic, second pulmonic, tricuspid, and mitral areas.

Female Breasts

- Inspect in these positions—patient's arms hanging loosely at the sides, extended over head or flexed behind the neck, pushing hands on hips, hands pushed together in front of chest, patient leaning forward.
- Perform chest wall sweep and bimanual digital palpation.
- Palpate axillary, supraclavicular, and infraclavicular lymph nodes (if not already performed).

Male Breasts

- Inspect breasts and nipples for symmetry, enlargement, surface characteristics.
- Palpate breast tissue.
- Palpate axillary, supraclavicular, and infraclavicular lymph nodes.

PATIENT RECLINING 45 DEGREES

- Assist patient to a reclining position at a 45-degree angle. Stand to side of patient that allows greatest comfort and approach for examination.
- Inspect chest in recumbent position.
- Inspect jugular venous pulsations; measure right jugular venous pressure.

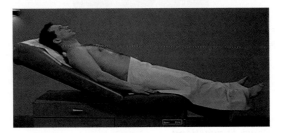

PATIENT SUPINE, CHEST EXPOSED

Assist patient into supine position. If patient cannot tolerate lying flat, maintain head elevation at 30-degree angle. Uncover chest while keeping abdomen and lower extremities draped.

Female Breasts

- Inspect and palpate with patient in recumbent position. Use light, medium, and deep palpation with patient's arm over her head.
- Depress nipple into well behind the areola.

Heart

- Palpate chest wall for thrills, heaves, pulsations.
- Auscultate systematically; turn patient slightly to left side and repeat auscultation.

PATIENT SUPINE, ABDOMEN EXPOSED

Have patient remain supine. Cover chest with patient's gown. Arrange draping to expose abdomen from pubis to epigastrium.

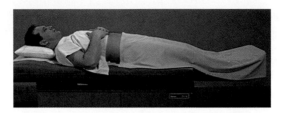

Abdomen

- Inspect skin characteristics, contour, pulsations, movement.
- Auscultate all quadrants for bowel sounds.
- Auscultate aorta and renal, iliac, and femoral arteries for bruits or venous hums.
- Percuss all quadrants for tone.
- Percuss liver borders and estimate span.
- Percuss left midaxillary line for splenic dullness.
- Lightly palpate all quadrants.
- Deeply palpate all quadrants.
    - Palpate right costal margin for liver border.
    - Palpate left costal margin for spleen.
    - Palpate at the flanks for right and left kidneys.
    - Palpate midline for aortic pulsation.
- Test abdominal reflexes.
- Have patient raise head as you inspect abdominal muscles.

Inguinal Area
- Palpate for lymph nodes, pulses, hernias.

External Genitalia, Males
- Inspect penis, urethral meatus, scrotum, pubic hair.
- Palpate scrotal contents.
- Test cremasteric reflex.

PATIENT SUPINE, LEGS EXPOSED

Have patient remain supine. Arrange drapes to cover abdomen and pubis, and to expose lower extremities.

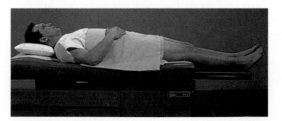

Feet and Legs

- Inspect for skin characteristics, hair distribution, muscle mass, musculo-skeletal configuration.
- Palpate for temperature, texture, edema, pulses (dorsalis pedis, posterior tibial, popliteal).
- Test range of motion and strength of toes, feet, ankles, knees.

Hips

- Palpate hips for stability.
- Test range of motion and strength of hips.

PATIENT SITTING, LAP DRAPED

Assist patient to a sitting position. Have patient wear gown with a drape across lap.

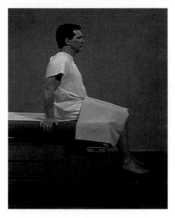

Musculoskeletal

- Observe patient moving from lying to sitting position.
- Note coordination, use of muscles, ease of movement.

Neurologic

- Test sensory function—dull and sharp sensation of forehead, cheeks, chin, lower arms, hands, lower legs, feet.
- Test position sense and vibratory sensation of wrists, ankles.
- Test two-point discrimination of palms, thighs, back.
- Test stereognosis, graphesthesia.
- Test fine motor function, coordination, and position sense of upper extremities, asking patient to do the following:
  - Touch nose with alternating index fingers.

- Rapidly alternate touching fingers to thumb.
- Rapidly move index finger between own nose and examiner's finger.
- Test fine motor function, coordination, and position sense of lower extremities, asking patient to do following:
  - Run heel down tibia of opposite leg.
- Test deep tendon reflexes and compare bilaterally—biceps, triceps, brachioradial, patellar, Achilles.
- Test plantar reflex bilaterally.

PATIENT STANDING

Assist patient to standing position. Stand next to patient.

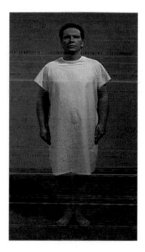

Spine
- Inspect and palpate spine as patient bends over at waist.
- Test range of motion—hyperextension, lateral bending, rotation of upper trunk.

Neurologic
- Observe gait.
- Test proprioception and cerebellar function:
  - Perform Romberg test.
  - Ask patient to walk heel to toe.
  - Ask patient to stand on one foot, then the other, with eyes closed.
  - Ask patient to hop in place on one foot, then other, with eyes open.

Abdominal/Genital
- Test for inguinal and femoral hernias.

FEMALE PATIENT, LITHOTOMY POSITION

Assist female patient into lithotomy position and drape appropriately. Examiner is seated.

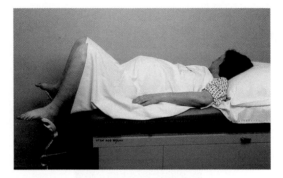

External Genitalia
- Inspect pubic hair, labia, clitoris, urethral opening, vaginal opening, perineal and perianal area, anus.
- Palpate labia and Bartholin glands; milk Skene glands.

Internal Genitalia
- Perform speculum examination:
  - Inspect vagina and cervix.
  - Collect Pap smear/human papillomavirus and other necessary specimens.
- Perform bimanual palpation to assess for characteristics of vagina, cervix, uterus, adnexa (examiner standing).
- Perform rectovaginal examination to assess rectovaginal septum, broad ligaments.
- Perform rectal examination:
  - Assess anal sphincter tone and surface characteristics; palpate circumferentially for rectal mass.
  - Obtain rectal culture if needed.
  - Note characteristics of stool when gloved finger is removed. Test for occult blood.

MALE PATIENT, BENDING FORWARD

- Assist male patient in leaning over examining table (or into knee-chest or lateral decubitus position). Stand behind patient.
- Inspect sacrococcygeal and perianal areas.
- Perform rectal examination:
  - Palpate sphincter tone and surface characteristics.
  - Obtain rectal culture if needed.
  - Palpate prostate gland and seminal vesicles.
  - Note characteristics of stool when gloved finger is removed. Test for occult blood.

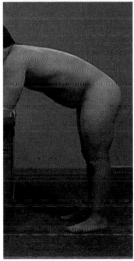

CONCLUSION

- Allow patient to dress in private.
- Share findings and interpretations with patient.
- Answer the patient's additional questions.
- Confirm that the patient has a clear understanding of all aspects of the situation.
- If patient is examined in a hospital bed:
  - Put everything back in order when finished.
  - Make sure patient is comfortably settled in an appropriate manner.
  - Put bed side rails up if clinical condition warrants it.
  - Make sure buttons and buzzers are within easy reach.

CHAPTER 21

Age-Specific Examination: Infants, Children, and Adolescents

EXAMINATION GUIDELINES

A pediatric physical examination must, of course, be age and developmentally appropriate. Not every observation and examination maneuver must be made on every child at every examination. What you do depends on the individual circumstance and your clinical judgment, each step dependent on the patient's age, physical condition, and emotional state. The order of the examination can and should be modified according to need. There is no one right way. The safety of the child on the examining table must be ensured. During most of infancy and into the pre–elementary school years (and even later), an adult's lap is most often a more secure surface for much and often all of the examination.

- Your notes should include a description of the child's behavior and the nature of the relationship during interactions with parent (or caregiver) and with you.
- Offer toys or paper and crayons to entertain child (if age appropriate), to develop rapport, and to evaluate development and neurologic status. Attempt to gain child's cooperation, even if it takes more time; future visits will be more pleasant for both of you.
- Only if absolutely necessary, restrain child for funduscopic, otoscopic, oral examinations; restraint is easier on an adult lap with the aid of the adult.
- Lessen fear of these examinations by permitting child to handle instruments, blow out light, or use them on a doll, a parent, or yourself.
- Take and record temperature, weight, length, or height; also take blood pressure (record extremity or extremities used, size of cuff, and method used).
- Note percentiles for all measurements, including body mass index for children ≥2 years.
- If clinical issues require it, include arm span, upper segment measurement (crown to top of symphysis), lower segment measurement (symphysis to soles of feet), upper/lower segment ratio, and chest circumference.
- Review parent-completed developmental screening tool to assess language, motor abilities, and social skills.
- Evaluate mental status as child interacts with you and parent.

CHILD PLAYING

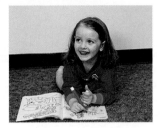

- While child plays on the floor, evaluate musculoskeletal and neurologic system while developing a rapport with child.
- Observe child's spontaneous activities.
- Ask child to demonstrate skills: turning pages in a book, building block towers, drawing geometric figures, coloring.
- Evaluate gait, jumping, hopping, range of motion.
- Muscle strength: Observe child climbing on parent's lap, stooping, and recovering.

CHILD ON PARENT'S LAP

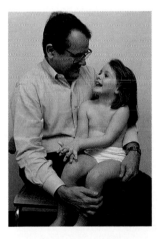

- Perform examination on parent's lap; the adult and the patient generally enjoy the experience more, and you, sitting on a stool, preferably with your eyes at the child's eye level, will find it easier than the examining table.
- Begin with child sitting and undressed except for diaper or underpants.

Upper Extremities
- Inspect arms for movement, size, shape, and skin lesions; observe use of hands; inspect hands for number and configuration of fingers, palmar creases.

- Palpate radial pulses.
- Elicit biceps and triceps reflexes.
- Take blood pressure at this point or later.

Lower Extremities

- Child may stand for much or part of examination.
- Inspect legs for movement, size, shape, alignment, lesions.
- Inspect feet for alignment, longitudinal arch, number of toes.
- Palpate femoral and dorsalis pedis pulses.
- Elicit plantar, Achilles, and patellar reflexes.

Head and Neck

- Inspect head.
- Inspect shape, alignment with neck, hairline, eyelids, palpebral folds, conjunctivae, sclerae, irides, position of auricles.
- Palpate anterior fontanel for size (age appropriate); head for sutures, depressions; hair for texture.
- Measure head circumference (up to age 36 months).
- Inspect neck for webbing, voluntary movement.
- Palpate neck: thyroid, muscle tone, lymph nodes, position of trachea.

Chest, Heart, Lungs

- Inspect chest for respiratory movement, size, shape, precordial movement, deformity, nipple and breast development.
- Palpate anterior chest, locate point of maximal impulse.
- Auscultate anterior, lateral, and posterior chest for breath sounds; count respirations.
- Auscultate all cardiac listening areas for S_1 and S_2, splitting, murmurs; count apical pulse.

CHILD RELATIVELY SUPINE, STILL ON LAP, DIAPER LOOSENED

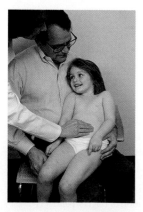

- Inspect abdomen.
- Auscultate for bowel sounds.
- Palpate: Identify size of liver and any other palpable organs or masses.
- Percuss.
- Palpate femoral pulses; compare with radial pulses.
- Palpate for inguinal lymph nodes.
- Inspect external genitalia.
- Males: Palpate scrotum for descent of testes and other masses.

CHILD STANDING

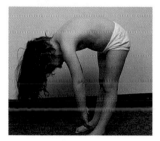

- Inspect spinal alignment as child bends slowly forward to touch toes.
- Observe posture from anterior, posterior, lateral views.
- Observe gait.

CHILD ON PARENT'S LAP

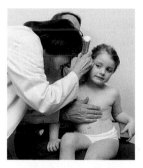

The following steps, often delayed to the end of the examination, are more easily performed with a child of appropriate age sitting on a parent's or caregiver's lap.
- Inspect eyes: pupillary light reflex, red reflex, corneal light reflex, extraocular movements, funduscopic examination.
- Perform otoscopic examination. Note position and description of pinnae.

- Inspect nasal mucosa.
- Inspect mouth and pharynx. Note number of teeth, deciduous or permanent, and any special characteristics.

NOTE: By the time child is of school age, it is usually possible to use an examination sequence very similar to that for adults.

AGE-SPECIFIC ANTICIPATED OBSERVATIONS AND GUIDELINES

Again, this is a suggested outline, always modified by human variation, and all percentages are subject to Gaussian distribution. History building can be facilitated by referring to baby books, report cards, pictures, and other materials the family may have at home.

2 WEEKS OF AGE

History (particular attention)
- Pertinent perinatal history
- Social: sleeping arrangements, housing
- Maternal mood and social support
- Stool pattern
- Umbilicus: healing, discharge, granulation
- Diet: feeding modality, schedule

Development
By this age:
- 80% will lift and turn head when in prone position.
- 40% will follow an object to midline visually.
- 35% will vocalize, become quiet in response to a voice.
- 45% will regard a face intently, diminishing activity for the moment.

Physical Examination (particular attention)
- Establish growth curves (weight, height, head circumference).
- Examine hips.
- Test reflexes: Moro, root, grasp, step.

Anticipatory Guidance (particular attention)
- Sleep (emphasize supine position and safe sleep environment)
- Feeding: use of pacifier (need to suck)
- Use of bulb syringe (nasal stuffiness)
- Safety: falling, crib, car seats
- Skin care
- Clothing
- Illness: temperature taking
- Crying (holding the baby)

Plans and Problems

- What risks have revealed themselves as you have gotten to know the family? What are apparent problems? Start a problem list and make appropriate dispositions.
- Review results of newborn metabolic screening.
- Consider immunization needs and, throughout, attempt to follow American Academy of Pediatrics guidelines; on each visit, discuss benefits, risks, and side effects of immunizations (always remember risks for the immunocompromised).

2 MONTHS OF AGE

History (particular attention)

- Expressions of parental concern
- Child's apparent temperament
- Sleep cycle
- Feeding patterns, frequency
- Stooling pattern, frequency, color, consistency, straining
- Social issues:
  Maternal mood
  Father's involvement
  Living conditions
  Smoking, other concerning environmental exposures
  Any apparent high-risk concerns

Development

By this age:
- Gross motor:
  80% will lift head to 45 degrees in prone position.
  45% will lift head to as much as 90 degrees in prone position.
  25% will roll over stomach to back.
- Fine motor:
  ≥99% will follow a moving object to midline.
  85% will follow a moving object past midline.
- Language:
  Almost all will diminish activity at the sound of a voice.
  35% will spontaneously vocalize.
  Many will vocalize responsively.
- Psychosocial:
  Almost all will diminish activity when regarding a face.
  Almost all will respond to a friendly, cooing face with a social smile.
  50% may smile spontaneously or even laugh aloud.

Physical Examination (particular attention)

- Growth curves (weight, height, head circumference)
- Hearing

- Vision
- Hips

Anticipatory Guidance

- Feeding (delay or at least downplay solids; avoid citrus, wheat, mixed foods, eggs; minimize water)
- When and if mother returns to work
- Hiccups
- Straining at stool
- Visual and auditory stimulus (mobiles, mirrors, rattles, singing and talking to baby)
- Sibling rivalry (if there are siblings or other children in home)
- Babysitters and other caregivers (checking references, reliability)
- Safety (rolling over, playpen, car seat, smoke detectors in home)
- Sleep (re-emphasize location and supine position)
- Smoking in home and contribution to poor health

Plans and Problems

- Review immunizations and provide as appropriate.
- List problems (e.g., allergies, medications, any areas of concern), and make appropriate plans and, if necessary, referrals.

4 MONTHS OF AGE

History (particular attention)

- Parental concerns
- Infant's sleep cycle and temperament
- Feeding patterns, frequency
- Stooling pattern, frequency, color, consistency, straining
- Social issues:
  Maternal mood
  Father's involvement
  Review family structure and social supports
  Smoking, other concerning environmental exposures
  Any apparent high-risk concerns

Development

By this age:
- Gross motor:
  80%, when prone, will lift chest up with arm support.
  80% will roll over from stomach to back.
  35% will have no head lag when pulled to sitting position, and many will then hold head steady when kept in that position.
- Fine motor:
  60% will reach for a dangling object.
  Almost all will bring hands together.
  Almost all will follow a face or object up to 180 degrees.

- Language:
  Almost all will laugh aloud.
  20% will appear to initiate vocalization.
- Psychosocial:
  80% will smile spontaneously.
  Many will regard their own hand for several seconds.

Physical Examination (particular attention)

- Update growth curves (weight, height, head circumference).
- Reassess hearing.
- Reassess vision.

Anticipatory Guidance

- Introduction of solid food (cereal)
- Stool changes with changes in diet
- Drooling and teething
- Thumb sucking, pacifiers, bottles at bedtime
- Safety (aspiration, rolling over, holding baby with hot liquids, re-emphasize earlier discussions [e.g., car seat])
- Re-emphasis on environmental stimulus
- Further discussion of babysitters and other caregivers
- Use of antipyretics (e.g., acetaminophen)

Plans and Problems

- Review immunizations and provide as appropriate.
- Maintain problem list, making appropriate plans and, if necessary, referrals.

6 MONTHS OF AGE

History (interim details)

- Parental concerns
- Sleep patterns
- Diet
- Stooling pattern
- Further exploration of social issues
- If either parent has not attended these care visits regularly, encourage his or her participation and address relevant issues.

Development

By this age:

- Gross motor:
  90%, pulled to a sitting position, will have no head lag.
  60% will sit alone.
  75% will bear some weight on legs.
  Almost all will roll over.

- Fine motor:
  More than half will pass a toy from hand to hand.
  60%, in a sitting position, will look for a toy.
  40%, in a sitting position, will take two cubes.
- Language:
  60% will turn toward a voice.
  30% will initiate speech sounds (e.g., "mama," "dada") but not specifically.
- Psychosocial:
  30% may cry and turn away from strangers.
  40% may put an object in mouth to explore it, may feed self.
  60% may resist an attempt to pull away an object while holding it.

Physical Examination (particular attention)
- Update growth curves.
- Double-check hearing and vision.
- Look for any new findings and recheck prior findings.

Anticipatory Guidance
- Bedtime routines (discuss putting child to bed while child is awake; waking up at night)
- Fear of strangers
- Separation anxiety
- Safety (begin discussions about what toddlers can get into, cabinets, hot water, electrical outlets, medications and other poisons; inform about local poison control center)
- Shoes, when and if to use them
- Teething, oral hygiene
- Offering a cup
- Checking fluoride intake
- Addition of solid foods

Plans and Problems
- Review immunizations and provide as appropriate.
- Consider need for a serum lead level, hemoglobin or hematocrit value.
- Maintain problem list, making appropriate plans and, if necessary, referrals.

9 MONTHS OF AGE

History (interim details)
- Parental concerns
- Continued attention to sleep, diet, stooling patterns
- Continuing attention to social issues

Development
By this age:
- Gross motor:
  Almost 100% will sit alone.
  80% will stand alone.
  45% will cruise.
  Some will have begun competent crawling.
- Fine motor:
  70% will have thumb-finger grasp.
  60% will bang two cubes together.
  Almost all will finger feed.
- Language:
  75% will imitate speech sounds.
  75% will use "mama," "dada" nonspecifically.
- Psychosocial:
  Almost 100% will try to get to a toy that is out of reach.
  85% will play repetitive games (e.g., peekaboo).
  45% will be shy with strangers and may cry.

Physical examination (particular attention)
- Update growth curves.
- Reassess earlier findings and note any new findings.

Anticipatory guidance
- Oral hygiene—for example, water without sugar in bottles (avoid tooth decay)
- Sleep and desirability of routine (naps, separation anxiety, and how to deal with it)
- Re-emphasis on checking references and reliability of babysitters and caregivers
- Safety—for example, stair gates and toddlers, falls, poisoning, burns, aspiration (never enough emphasis on safety, smoking in the home, etc.)
- Weaning, breast and/or bottle
- Uses of discipline

Plans and Problems
- Review immunizations and provide as appropriate.
- Perform developmental screening (using parent-administered validated tool).
- Consider need for a serum lead level, hemoglobin or hematocrit value.
- Maintain problem list, making appropriate plans and, if necessary, referrals.

12 MONTHS OF AGE
History (interim details)
- Assess parental concerns.
- Reassess social and system review.

Development
By this age:
- Gross motor:
  85% will cruise.
  70% will stand alone briefly.
  50% will walk to some extent, and more will try it with hands held.
- Fine motor:
  90% will bang two cubes together.
  70% will have a good pincer grasp.
- Language:
  80% will use "mama" and "dada" specifically.
  30% will use as many as three additional words.
  Almost all will indulge in immature jargoning.
- Psychosocial:
  Almost all will respond to parent's presence and voice.
  Almost all will wave bye-bye.
  85% will play pat-a-cake.
  50% will drink from a cup.
  About half, perhaps a bit more, will play ball with examiner.

Physical Examination (particular attention)
- Update growth curves.
- Continue reassessment.
- Evaluate gait if walking has begun.

Anticipatory Guidance
- Reduced food intake in many (this is expected)
- Weaning or eliminating bottle use (especially at night)
- Increased use of table food
- Dental health, toothbrushing
- Toilet training (expectations, attitudes)
- Discipline (e.g., limit setting)
- Safety (childproofing house, car, neighborhood, etc.)

Plans and Problems
- Review immunizations and provide as appropriate.
- Consider need for a serum lead level, hemoglobin or hematocrit value, tuberculin test.
- Maintain problem list, making appropriate plans and, if necessary, referrals.

15 MONTHS OF AGE
History (interim details)
- Assess parental concerns.
- Reassess social and system review.

Development

By this age:

- Gross motor:

  Almost all will walk well.

  Almost all will stoop to recover an object.

  35% will walk up steps with help.

- Fine motor:

  Almost all will drink from a cup.

  Almost all will have a neat pincer grasp.

  70% will scribble with crayon.

  60% will make a tower with two cubes.

- Language:

  Almost all will use "mama" and "dada" specifically.

  75% will use as many as three additional words.

  30% will put two words together.

- Psychosocial:

  Many more than 50% will play ball with examiner.

  50% will try to use a spoon.

  45% will try to remove clothing.

Physical Examination (particular attention)

- Update growth curves.
- Continue reassessment.
- Evaluate gait.

Anticipatory Guidance

- Negativism and independence
- Dental health (visit to a dentist)
- Toilet training
- Weaning
- Discipline (e.g., need for consistency)
- Safety (all issues, repetitively)

Plans and Problems

- Review immunizations and provide as appropriate.
- Consider need for a serum lead level, hemoglobin or hematocrit value, tuberculin test.
- Maintain problem list, making appropriate plans and, if necessary, referrals.

18 MONTHS OF AGE

History (interim details)

- Assess parental concerns.
- Reassess social and system review.

Development

By this age:
- Gross motor:
  55% will have begun to walk up stairs without much help.
  70% will have started to walk backward.
  More than that will have tried running with at least some success.
  45% will have tried with some success to kick a ball forward, given the opportunity.
- Fine motor:
  80% will scribble if given a crayon.
  80% will make a tower with two cubes.
  About half of those will attempt with some success a tower of as many as four cubes.
- Language:
  Almost all will have mature jargoning.
  85% will have at least three words in addition to "mama" and "dada."
  Many of those will put two words together.
  More than half will respond to a one-step command (e.g., when asked to point to a body part).
- Psychosocial:
  Well more than half will assist with taking off their clothes.
  75% will use a spoon successfully, albeit with some spillage.

Physical Examination (particular attention)

- Update growth curves.
- Continue reassessment; search for new findings.
- Continue to evaluate gait.

Anticipatory Guidance

- Sleep (location, naps, nightmares)
- Diet (mealtime battles)
- Dental health (toothbrushing, dentist)
- Toilet training
- Discipline (methods and, again, consistency)
- Safety (never enough discussion [e.g., car seat, childproofing home])
- Self-comforting (masturbation, thumb sucking, favorite blankets and toys)
- Child care settings if one is necessary

Plans and Problems

- Review immunizations and provide as appropriate.
- Perform developmental and autism screening (using parent-administered validated tools).
- Consider need for serum lead level, hemoglobin or hematocrit value, tuberculin test.
- Maintain problem list, making appropriate plans and, if necessary, referrals.

2 YEARS OF AGE

History (interim details)
- Assess parental concerns.
- Reassess social and system review.

Development
By this age:
- Gross motor:
  All should run well.
  All should walk up steps of reasonable height without holding on.
  90% will kick a ball forward.
  80% will throw a ball overhand.
  60% will do a little jump.
  40% may balance on one foot for 1 to 2 seconds.
- Fine motor:
  Almost all should scribble with a pencil.
  90% will make a tower of four cubes.
  70% will copy a vertical line.
- Language:
  All should point to and name parts of body.
  85% will readily combine two different words.
  80% will understand on and under.
  75% will name a picture.
- Psychosocial:
  85% will give a toy to mother or other significant person.
  60% will put on some clothing alone and, often, also remove a garment.
  50% will play games with others.

Physical Examination (particular attention)
- Update growth curves.
- Continue reassessment; note new findings.
- Examine mouth and count number of teeth.

Anticipatory Guidance
- Independence (limit setting, temper tantrums)
- Peer interaction
- Safety (poisons and potential poisons, water temperature, car safety seat use)
- Toilet training
- Nightmares
- Use of a cup for drinking (as much as possible)

Plans and Problems
- Review immunizations and provide as appropriate.
- Perform developmental screening (using parent-administered validated tool).

- Consider need for serum lead level, hemoglobin or hematocrit value, dental referral, tuberculin test.
- Maintain problem list, making appropriate plans and, if necessary, referrals.

3 YEARS OF AGE

History (interim details)

- Assess parental concerns.
- Reassess social and system review.

Development

By this age:

- Gross motor:
  75% will balance on one foot for at least 1 second.
  75% will negotiate a successful broad jump.
  40% will balance on one foot for as long as 5 seconds.
- Fine motor:
  80% will copy a circle in addition to a vertical line.
  80% will build a tower of as many as eight cubes.
- Language:
  Speech is becoming more clearly understood in more than half.
  80% will use plurals appropriately.
  Almost half will give their first and last names appropriately.
- Psychosocial:
  90% will put on clothing alone.
  75% will play interactive games.
  50% will separate from mother or other significant person without too much stress.
  Many will have begun to wash and dry hands.

Physical Examination (particular attention)

- Update growth curves.
- Continue reassessment; note new findings.
- Assess whether teeth are coming in appropriately.

Anticipatory Guidance

- Degrees of independence (limit setting and encouragement, a fine balance), other aspects of discipline
- Safety (car seat, guns in the home, strangers)
- Personal hygiene (handwashing, toothbrushing, proper use of toilet tissue)
- Daycare

Plans and Problems

- Review immunizations and provide as appropriate.
- Conduct formal vision screening.

- Consider need for serum lead level, hemoglobin or hematocrit value, tuberculin test.
- Maintain problem list, making appropriate plans and, if necessary, referrals.

4 YEARS OF AGE

History (interim details)
- Assess parental concerns.
- Reassess social and system review.

Development
By this age:
- Gross motor:
  75% will hop on one foot.
  75% will balance on one foot for as long as 5 seconds.
  65% will be able to imitate a heel-toe walk.
  Many will have begun to throw overhand.
- Fine motor:
  Almost all will copy a circle and a plus sign.
  80% will pick longer line of two.
  50% will begin to draw a person in three parts.
- Language:
  Speech is quite understandable in almost all.
  95% will give their first and last names.
  85% will understand cold, tired, hungry.
  80% will identify three of four colors.
- Psychosocial:
  Almost all will play games with other children.
  70% will dress without supervision.

Physical Examination (particular attention)
- Update growth curves.
- Continue reassessment; note new findings.
- Remind that hearing and vision must be evaluated at each visit.
- Remind that taking blood pressure is an integral part of physical examination.

Anticipatory Guidance
- Importance of reading to child frequently
- Need for a booster seat in the car
- Fears and fantasies
- Separation (reliance on other adults as time goes by)
- Safety (matches and lighters out of reach, strangers, street, window guards)
- Personal hygiene (again, importance of frequent toothbrushing)

Plans and Problems
- Review immunizations and provide as appropriate.
- Conduct formal hearing and vision screening.
- Consider need for serum lead level, hemoglobin or hematocrit value.
- Maintain problem list, making appropriate plans and, if necessary, referrals.

5 YEARS OF AGE
History (interim details)
- Assess parental concerns.
- Reassess social and system review.

Development
By this age:
- Gross motor:
  Almost all will hop nicely on one foot.
  75% will balance on one foot for as long as 10 seconds.
  60% will do a heel-toe walk backward reasonably well.
- Fine motor:
  85% will draw a person in three parts.
  65% will draw a person in as many as six parts.
  60% will copy a square.
- Language:
  Almost all will identify four colors.
  Almost all will understand on, under, in front of, behind.
  More than half will define adequately five of the following eight words—
      ball, cake, desk, house, banana, curtain, fence, ceiling.
- Psychosocial:
  Almost all will dress without supervision.
  Almost all will brush teeth without help.
  Almost all will play board and card games.
  Almost all will be relaxed when left with a babysitter.
  More than half will prepare their own cereal.

Physical Examination (particular attention)
- Update growth curves.
- Continue reassessment; note new findings.

Anticipatory Guidance
- Reading together
- School readiness (plays with others, endures separation from parents)
- Chores
- Discipline (consistency, praising)
- Sex identification, education

- Peer interaction
- Television
- Safety (booster seat, guns in home, bike helmets, pool safety)

It is not usually possible to cover so many topics at one visit, so it is usually necessary to be selective based on your knowledge of the family situation.

Plans and Problems

- Review immunizations and provide as appropriate.
- Consider need for a tuberculin test.
- Maintain problem list, making appropriate plans and, if necessary, referrals.

ELEMENTARY SCHOOL YEARS (6-12 YEARS OF AGE)

History (interim details)

- Parental concerns
- Child's concerns
- Reassess social and system review
- Attention span
- Behavior at home and in school
- School accomplishments and experience
- Enuresis, encopresis, constipation, nightmares

Development

By this time gross and fine motor problems have most often become apparent (but not always; neurologic examination should not be shortchanged). Language and psychosocial skills can be readily investigated in talks with parents and child, and in explorations of school and play experiences. Socialization and developing maturity may have different expressions at home, on the playground, and in school, and when with people of different ages and different degrees of acquaintance. Talks with teachers, report cards, and various drawings and other efforts that the child brings home from school can be very helpful.

Physical Examination (particular attention)

- Update growth curves.
- Continue reassessment; note new findings.
- Begin Tanner stage assessment.

Anticipatory Guidance

- Parent–child rapport
- Need for praise
- Responsibility
- Safety (booster seat and seat belt use, guns in the home, fire safety, bike helmets, pool safety)

- Allowance
- Television
- Sex education
- Dental care
- Adult supervision
- Discipline (limit setting)

Again, time constraints almost always make it necessary to adjust the menu for anticipatory guidance to your judgment about the family's needs.

Plans and Problems
- Review immunizations and provide as appropriate.
- Consider need for a tuberculin test.
- Consider dyslipidemia screening,
- Maintain problem list, making appropriate plans and, if necessary, referrals.

ADOLESCENTS

We have assumed a continuing relationship with the patient from birth on. If you are seeing a patient for the first time, begin with a full history and physical examination.

History (interim details)
- Patient's concerns
- Parental concerns
- Menstrual history
- Use of tobacco, alcohol, recreational drugs
- Diet and exercise
- Sexual activity (relationships, partner violence, pregnancy and contraceptive use); exact timing for all of this should rely on your assessment of the situation and your judgment; in general, social experience
- School experience
- Suicidal ideation; always be on the alert, and bring it up when necessary
- Update knowledge of home and family structure

An adolescent patient (and some elementary-school children) may prefer to be or should be seen alone at times and as they get older, most often or always. This does not mean, however, that the parents are not involved. Proper balance in this relies on your judgment.

Development

By this time adolescent's physical, neurologic, and cognitive abilities should be well understood, but nothing should be taken for granted. Conversation with patient, parent or parents, and teachers; school records; and, of course, a careful physical examination should all be helpful.

Physical Examination (particular attention)
- Update growth curves.
- Continue reassessment; note new findings.
- Tanner stage assessment.
- Assess spinal curvatures, particularly in early-adolescent female patients.

Anticipatory Guidance
- Puberty and its issues; body image
- Sexuality, sexually transmitted infections, contraception
- Diet
- Tobacco, alcohol, drugs
- Risk-taking behavior
- Exercise
- Safety (guns in the home, seat-belt use, bike helmets)
- Family and other social relationships
- Independence and responsibility
- School and the future

Time constraints almost always make it necessary to adjust the menu for anticipatory guidance to your judgment about the adolescent's and/or the family's needs.

Plans and Problems
- Review immunizations and provide as appropriate.
- Consider need for tuberculin test, sexually transmitted infection screening, hemoglobin or hematocrit determination, dyslipidemia screening.
- Maintain problem list, making appropriate plans and, if necessary, referrals.

CHAPTER 22

Age-Specific Examination: Special Populations and Older Adults

EXAMINATION GUIDELINES

Variability exists in knowledge, experience, cognitive abilities, and personality among patients. These differences can affect your interaction. Persons with disabilities and older adults may experience some decline in their abilities, and these changes may not all occur at the same rate. Adaptation to patients' needs with disabling physical, intellectual, or emotional states (e.g., acute disabling illness, deafness, blindness, depression, psychosis, developmental delays, or neurologic impairments) is necessary.

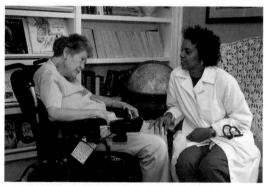

Interviewing a patient with a physical disability. Note the uncluttered surroundings; be sure the patient in a wheelchair has room to maneuver.

Some patients may have sensory losses, such as hearing, that make communication more difficult. Position yourself so that the patient can see your face. Speak clearly and slowly; shouting magnifies the problem by distorting consonants and vowels. For deaf patients who use sign language, use of a sign language interpreter is best. Impaired vision and difficulties with light-dark adaptation are a problem with written interview forms. Large print and lighting that does not glare or reflect in the eyes or individualized assistance is helpful.

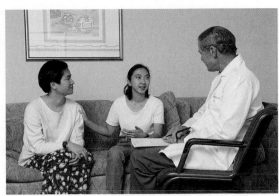

Interviewing a patient with the help of an interpreter. Someone other than a family member should act as interpreter to bridge the language difference between the health care provider and the patient.

The patient has most often learned the best way to be transferred from a wheelchair or bed to another site or to a different position. Consult patient about this.

Let a hearing-, speech-, or vision-impaired patient guide you to the best communication system for your mutual purposes.

Bowel and bladder concerns are common to many individuals with disabilities and should be given the necessary attention during the examination process.

COGNITIVE ASSESSMENT

Some older adults or individuals with intellectual delay may be confused or experience memory loss, particularly for recent events. Take whatever extra time is needed. Ask short (but not leading) questions, and keep your language simple. Consult other family members to clarify discrepancies or to fill in the gaps. When necessary, use other health care professionals involved in care and the patient's record as resources for a more complete background.

Mental status is assessed continuously throughout the entire interaction with a patient by evaluating the patient's alertness, orientation, cognitive abilities, and mood. Observe the patient's physical appearance, behavior, and responses to questions asked during the history (see figure, p. 276). Evaluate the patient's mental status throughout the encounter (see Chapter 3).

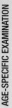

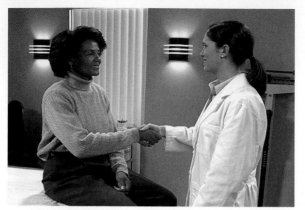

During the initial greeting, observe the patient for behavior, emotional status, grooming, and body language. Note the patient's body posture and ability to make eye contact.

TESTING MEMORY IN VISUALLY IMPAIRED PATIENTS

When a patient is visually impaired, test recent memory with unrelated words rather than observed objects. Pick four unrelated words that sound distinctly different, such as "green," "daffodil," "hero," and "sofa" or "bird," "carpet," "treasure," and "orange." Tell the patient to remember these words. After 5 minutes, ask the patient to list the four words.

Cognitive impairment that deprives ability to join in decision-making processes underscores the need for advance directives, which document the patient's wishes regarding extraordinary means of life support (e.g., ventilation assistance and feeding tubes). These documents should be complemented by a surrogate (e.g., spouse, child, sibling, or other person with a close relationship) who has a legally executed durable power of attorney for health care.

Multiple problems that require multiple medications increase risk for iatrogenic disorders and issues related to interactions. A medication history with attention to interactions of drugs, diseases, and aging is needed for prescribed and over-the-counter medications and herbal preparations.

Aging, disability, a debilitating illness, and the onset of frailty increase dependency on others, worry about tomorrow, and grieving for what has been lost. Recognize these vast concerns and the sense of loss in both the patient and the immediate caregiver. Maintaining function is a compelling concern of older adults.

FUNCTIONAL ASSESSMENT

Functional assessment is an evaluation of a patient's ability to achieve the basic activities of daily living (ADLs). Questions concerning the ability to take care of one's daily needs are part of the review of systems.

Activities of Daily Living

The ability to perform instrumental ADLs, or the ability to live independently, is an important assessment. Determine the patient's ability to perform the following:

ADLs Assessment

Shop, cook, and prepare nutritious meals
Use problem-solving skills
Manage medications (purchase, understand, and follow directions)
Manage personal finances and business affairs
Speak, write, and understand spoken and written language
Remember appointments, family occasions, holidays, household tasks

The personal and social history should include other dimensions of functional capacity such as social, spiritual, and economic resources; recreational activity; sleep patterns; environmental control; and use of the health care system.

Functional assessment should be given to anyone limited by disease or disability and includes:

Functional Assessment

Mobility	Upper extremity function
Difficulty walking standard distances: ½ mile, 2 to 3 blocks, ⅓ block, across a room	Difficulty grasping small objects, opening jars
Difficulty climbing stairs, up and down	Difficulty reaching out or up overhead, such as to take something off a shelf
Problems with balance	
Housework	**Instrumental ADLs**
Heavy (vacuuming, scrubbing floors)	Bathing
Light (dusting)	Dressing
Meal preparation	Toileting
Shopping	Moving from bed to chair, chair to standing
	Eating
	Walking in home

Any limitations will affect a patient's independence and autonomy, and increase reliance on other people and on assistive devices.

In older patients, these limitations indicate the loss of physical reserve and the potential loss of physical function and independence that indicate the onset of frailty.

Characteristics of Fraility

Weight loss	Weakness
Diminished ability to respond to stress	Low activity

Frailty is an at-risk state caused by the age-associated accumulation of deficits. With multisystem dysregulation, decreased physiologic reserves, and increased vulnerability to stressors, frailty shares features of normal aging (Fedarko, 2011; Rockwood and Mitnitski, 2011), but age and frailty are not necessarily synonymous.

CHAPTER 23

The Healthy Female Evaluation

Following are items to consider for inclusion as part of a routine female health examination or well-woman visit. This is not intended as an all-inclusive list. Some items may vary depending on the woman's age, health status, and particular risk factors. Medical history and review of systems may also be indicated. Age and risk-status guidelines for preventive services are available from a variety of sources and authorities.*

HISTORY

HISTORY OF PRESENT ILLNESS

- Age
- Last normal menstrual period
- Menopause—age achieved, symptoms
- Obstetric history—number of pregnancies, term pregnancies, preterm pregnancies, abortions/miscarriages, living children (GTPAL)
- Contraceptive measures and history
- Sexual history
- Breast lumps, discharge, pain, skin changes
- Unusual vaginal bleeding or discharge
- Abdominal or pelvic pain or bloating
- Urinary symptoms

RISK ASSESSMENT

- Cardiovascular—smoking, hypertension, diet, body mass index (BMI), exercise, family history
- Cancer—personal/family history of breast, ovarian, or colon cancer; history of sun exposure
- Infection—sexually transmitted infection (STI) exposure; tuberculosis exposure; hepatitis vaccine or exposure; tetanus/flu immunization
- Metabolic—calcium supplement, family/personal history of osteoporosis; exercise; personal/family history of diabetes mellitus; hearing impairment in older adults

---

*Authorities that produce prevention guidelines include Academy of Family Physicians, American Cancer Society, American College of Obstetricians and Gynecologists, American College of Physicians, American Geriatrics Society, Canadian Task Force on the Periodic Health Examination, National Cancer Institute, and U.S. Preventive Services Task Force.

- Injury—alcohol, seat belts, guns, family/partner violence
- Mental health—depression: vegetative symptoms (eating, sleeping, concentration, energy, social interaction)

HEALTH HABITS

- Breast self-awareness
- Pap smear—how often; date of last Pap smear; results, ever an abnormal result?
- Human papillomavirus (HPV) test—date, results
- Mammogram—date, result of last mammogram
- Diet—proportion of fat, protein, carbohydrate; calcium, vitamin D
- Exercise—amount, frequency
- Smoking/tobacco use—type, amount, frequency
- Alcohol/drug use—type, amount, frequency

PHYSICAL EXAMINATION

- Vital signs: blood pressure
- Height and weight; BMI
- Skin—lesions, moles
- Respiratory—rate, pattern, additional sounds
- Cardiovascular—rate, rhythm, regularity, additional sounds
- Peripheral vascular—pulses, edema, clubbing
- Breasts—contour, masses, nipple discharge, skin changes
- Lymph—regional lymphadenopathy (infraclavicular and supraclavicular, axillary, inguinal)
- Abdomen—bowel sounds, masses, organ enlargement, hernias
- Pelvic—lesions, discharge; Bartholin glands, urethra, Skene glands; vagina, cervix, adnexa, uterus; rectovaginal septum
- Rectal—hemorrhoids, masses, lesions

SCREENING RECOMMENDATIONS

- Cardiovascular
  Blood pressure—begin at age 18
  Lipid profile—begin at age 45
- Cancer
  Cervical: Pap smear/HPV testing:
  - Women aged 21 to 29 years: Pap test every 3 years. HPV testing should not be used in this age group unless it is needed after an abnormal Pap test result.
  - Women aged 30 and 65 years: Pap test plus an HPV test every 5 years or Pap test alone every 3 years.
  - Women older than 65 years at average risk who have had regular cervical cancer testing with normal results should not be tested. Once

testing is stopped, it should not be started again. Women with a history of a serious cervical precancer (cervical intraepithelial neoplasia grade 2 or 3) should continue to be tested for at least 20 years after that diagnosis, even if testing continues past age 65 years.

- Women with uterus and cervix removed for reasons not related to cervical cancer and who have no history of cervical cancer or serious precancer should not be tested.
- Women vaccinated against HPV should follow the screening recommendations for her age group.

Breast

- Clinical breast examination—younger than 40 years: every 3 years; older than 40 years: annually
- Screening mammogram—annually beginning at age 40 years; earlier if at increased risk; frequency depends on personal and family history and past results

Colorectal: begin age 50 years. Options are:

- Tests that detect adenomatous polyps and cancer
  - Flexible sigmoidoscopy every 5 years
  - Colonoscopy every 10 years
  - Double-contrast barium enema every 5 years
  - Computed tomography colography every 5 years
- Tests that primarily detect cancer
  - Annual guaiac-based fecal occult blood test with high test sensitivity
  - Annual fecal immunochemical test with high test sensitivity
  - Stool DNA test with high sensitivity (testing interval uncertain)
- Infection

  STI testing—depending on exposure status; chlamydia screening— all sexually active women age 25 or younger and women over age 25 with risk factors (e.g., women with a new or more than one sex partner); gonorrhea and syphilis screening—all sexually active women at increased risk

  TB skin testing—depending on risk status
- Metabolic

  BMI: obesity

  Fasting plasma glucose for diabetes type 2 in asymptomatic adults with sustained blood pressure (either treated or untreated) greater than 135/80 mm Hg

  Bone density—women ≥65 years; begin earlier in women whose fracture risk is equal to or greater than that of a 65-year-old white woman who has no additional risk factors

  Hearing impairment—older adults
- Injury

  Intimate partner violence (see Appendix Special Histories)
- Mental health

  Alcohol and substance abuse (see Appendix Special Histories)

CHAPTER 24

Sports Participation Evaluation

The overall goal of the preparticipation physical evaluation (PPE) is to ensure safe participation in an appropriate physical activity and not to restrict participation unnecessarily. Whether athletes receive the PPE in the context of an ongoing primary care relationship or as a focused preseason checkup, the following goals of the evaluation are universal:

- To identify conditions that may interfere with a person's ability to participate in a sport
- To identify health problems that increase the risk for injury or death during sports participation
- To help select an appropriate sport for a person's particular abilities and physical status

Sports and disciplined physical effort enhance fitness and coordination, increase self-esteem, and provide positive social experiences for participants, including individuals with physical and intellectual disabilities. Few children and youth have conditions that might limit participation, and most of these conditions are known before the PPE takes place. The PPE should be completed well enough in advance of the planned sports activity so that any needed specialist evaluations, rehabilitation, or therapy can be completed before participation begins. As a general rule, 6 weeks before participation is an appropriate time.

EXAMINATION GUIDELINES

Recommended components of the PPE include a focused medical history and examinations of high-yield areas, like the cardiac and orthopedic systems. Physical examination items are shown in italics in the following box.

Recommended Components of the PPE

General Medical History
- Illnesses or injuries since the last health visit or PPE
- History of having been denied or restricted from participation in sporting activities and reason for restriction
- History of heat illness or muscle cramps
- Current viral illness (patients with mononucleosis may return to play after 3 weeks if no longer symptomatic and no splenomegaly; fever at the time of the examination is an absolute contraindication because of the association with viral myocarditis)

Recommended Components of the PPE—cont'd

- Sickle cell trait or disease (adequate hydration is necessary, and caution should be taken to avoid extreme conditions because of the risk for rhabdomyolysis)
- Hospitalizations or surgeries
- All medications used by the athlete (including steroids and nutritional supplements or medications taken to enhance performance)
- Use of any special equipment or protective devices during sports participation
- Allergies (including food-, insect bite–, and exercise-provoked allergies), particularly those associated with anaphylaxis or respiratory compromise
- Absence of paired organs (single-organ athletes may participate if the single organ can be protected and the patient/caregivers understand the risks involved)
- Immunization status including hepatitis B, varicella, meningococcal, human papillomavirus, and pertussis
- *Height, weight, and body mass index*
- *Palpation of lymph nodes*

Cardiac
- Symptoms of exertional chest pain/discomfort
- Unexplained syncope/near-syncope
- Excessive exertional and unexplained dyspnea/fatigue, associated with exercise
- Prior recognition of a heart murmur
- *Elevated systemic blood pressure*
- Family history of premature death (sudden and unexpected, or otherwise) before age 50 years because of heart disease in one or more relatives
- Family history of disability from heart disease in a close relative younger than 50 years
- Specific knowledge of certain cardiac conditions in family members: hypertrophic or dilated cardiomyopathy, long QT syndrome or other ion channelopathies, Marfan syndrome, or clinically important arrhythmias
- *Heart murmur (auscultation should be performed in both supine and standing positions, or with Valsalva maneuver, to identify murmurs of dynamic left ventricular outflow obstruction); heart rate and rhythm to assess for arrhythmias*
- *Femoral pulses to exclude coarctation of the aorta*

Continued

SPORTS PARTICIPATION EVALUATION

Recommended Components of the PPE—cont'd

- *Physical stigmata of Marfan syndrome (e.g., arm span greater than height and hyperextensible joints)*
- *Brachial artery blood pressure (sitting position with appropriate size cuff, preferably taken in both arms)*

Respiratory
- Coughing, wheezing, or dyspnea with exercise
- Previous use of asthma medications
- Family history of asthma
- *Lung auscultation*

Neurologic
- History of a head injury with or without symptoms of a concussion (confusion, prolonged headache, memory problems)
- Numbness or tingling in the extremities
- Headaches
- History of seizure
- History of inability to move an extremity after a collision

Vision
- Visual problems
- Glasses or contact lenses
- Previous eye injuries
- *Visual acuity*

Orthopedic
- Previous injuries that have limited sports practice or participation
- Injuries that have been associated with pain, swelling, or the need for medical intervention
- Previous fractures or dislocated joints
- Previous or current use of a brace, orthotic, or other assistive device
- *Screening orthopedic examination*

Psychosocial
- Weight control and body image
- Dietary habits; calcium intake
- Stresses in personal life, at home, or in school
- Feelings of sadness, hopelessness, depression, or anxiety
- Use or abuse of recreational drugs, alcohol, tobacco, dietary or performance supplements
- *Attention to signs of eating disorders including oral ulcerations, decreased tooth enamel, edema*

Recommended Components of the PPE—cont'd

Genitourinary and Abdominal
- Age at menarche, last menstrual period, regularity of menstrual periods, number of periods in the last year, and longest interval between periods (athletic girls tend to experience menarche at a later age than nonathletic girls)
- *Palpation of the abdomen for organomegaly*
- *Palpation of the testicles*
- *Examination for inguinal hernias*

Dermatologic
- History of rashes, pressure sores, or other skin conditions
- History of boils or MRSA skin infections
- *Skin lesions suggestive of HSV, MRSA, or tinea corporis*

Adapted from Andrews, 1997, Maron et al, 2007, and 2010 Preparticipation Physical Evaluation History and Physical Examination Forms endorsed by the American Academy of Family Physicians, American Academy of Pediatrics, American College of Sports Medicine, American Medical Society for Sports Medicine, American Orthopedic Society for Sports Medicine, and the American Osteopathic Academy of Sports Medicine.

Garrick's "2-minute" 14-step orthopedic screening examination consists of observing the athlete in a variety of positions and postures that highlight asymmetries in range of motion, strength, and muscle bulk. These asymmetries serve to identify acute or old, poorly rehabilitated injuries. The steps shown in the figure on pp. 286-287 help in assessing most of the following:
- Posture and general muscle contour bilaterally
- Patient's duck walk, four steps with knees completely bent
- Spine for curvature and lumbar extension, fingers touching toes with knees straight
- Shoulder and clavicle for dislocation
- Neck, shoulders, elbows, forearms, hands, fingers, and hips for range of motion
- Knee ligaments for drawer sign

You should also assess the following:
- Gait
- Patient's ability to hop on each foot
- Patient's ability to walk on tiptoes and heels

Once a PPE has been completed, the health care provider can guide the patient with sport selection, plan therapy or rehabilitation of conditions or injuries, and in rare instances, discuss restrictions. The clinician may: (1) provide "clearance" for participation, (2) provide "clearance" for participation with recommendations for further evaluation and/or treatment, (3) restrict participation until further testing is performed, or (4) recommend complete

SPORTS PARTICIPATION EVALUATION

restriction from specific sports or all sports. Patients with findings from the PPE may require evaluation by a health care provider with appropriate knowledge and experience to assess the safety of a given sport for the athlete.

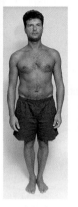

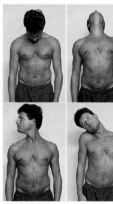

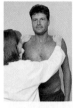

Step 3: Have the athlete shrug the shoulders against resistance from the examiner to evaluate trapezius strength.

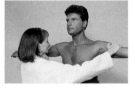

Step 1: Observe the standing athlete from the front for symmetry of trunk, shoulders, and extremities.

Step 2: Observe neck flexion, extension, lateral flexion on each side, and rotation to evaluate range of motion and the cervical spine.

Step 4: Have the athlete perform shoulder abduction against resistance from the examiner to assess deltoid strength.

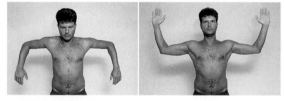

Step 5: Observe internal and external rotation of the shoulder to evaluate range of motion of the glenohumeral joint.

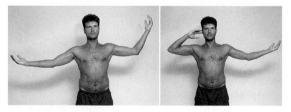

Step 6: Observe extension and flexion of the elbow to assess range of motion.

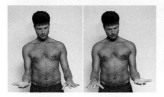

Step 7: Observe pronation and supination of the forearm to evaluate elbow and wrist range of motion.

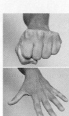

Step 8: Have the athlete clench the fist, then spread the fingers to assess range of motion in the hand and fingers.

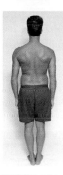

Step 9: Observe the standing athlete from the rear for symmetry of trunk, shoulders, and extremities.

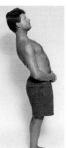

Step 10: Have the athlete stand with the knees straight and bend backward from the waist. Discomfort with extension of the lumbar spine may be associated with spondylolysis and spondylolisthesis.

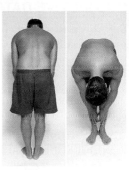

Step 11: Have the athlete stand with the knees straight and flex forward at the waist, first away from the examiner, then toward the examiner, to assess for scoliosis, spine range of motion, and hamstring flexibility.

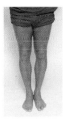

Step 12: Have the athlete stand facing the examiner with quadriceps flexed to observe symmetry of leg musculature.

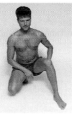

Step 13: Have the athlete duck walk four steps to assess hip, knee, and ankle range of motion, strength, and balance.

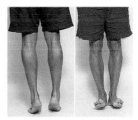

Step 14: Have the athlete stand on the toes, then the heels to evaluate calf strength, symmetry, and balance.

The 14-step screening orthopedic examination. The athlete should be dressed so that the joints and muscle groups included in the examination are easily visible, usually gym shorts for males and gym shorts and a T-shirt for females. Keep in mind that one of the most important points to look for in the orthopedic screening examination is symmetry.

SUBJECTIVE DATA—THE HISTORY

Subjective data are the positive and negative pieces of information that the patient offers. Record the patient's history, especially during an initial visit, to provide a comprehensive database. Arrange information appropriately in specific categories, usually in a particular sequence such as chronologic order with most recent information first. Include both positive and negative data that contribute to the assessment. Use the following organized sequence as a guide.

IDENTIFYING INFORMATION

Record data recommended by the health care facility.
- Patient's name
- Identification number/social security number
- Age, sex
- Marital status
- Address (home and business)
- Phone numbers
- Occupation, employer
- Insurance plan, number
- Date of visit
- For children and dependent adults, names of parents or next of kin
Put identifying information on each page of record.

SOURCE AND RELIABILITY OF INFORMATION

- Document who is providing the history and relationship to patient.
- Indicate when an old record is used.
- State judgment about reliability of information.

CHIEF CONCERN/PRESENTING PROBLEM/REASON FOR SEEKING CARE

Record a description of the patient's main reasons for seeking health care, in patient's own words with quotation marks. Paraphrase only if this makes the patient's concern more clear. Include duration of problem.

HISTORY OF PRESENT PROBLEM

- List and describe current symptoms of chief concern and their appearance chronologically in reverse order, dating events and symptoms.
- List any expected symptoms that are absent.
- Identify anyone in household with same symptoms.
- Note pertinent information from review of systems, family history, and personal/social history along with findings.
- Where more than one problem is identified, address each in a separate paragraph, including the following details of symptom occurrence:
  - Onset: when problem first started, chronologic order of events, setting and circumstances, manner of onset (sudden versus gradual)
  - Location: exact location, localized or generalized, radiation patterns
  - Duration: how long problem has lasted, intermittent or continuous, duration of each episode
  - Character: nature of symptom
  - Aggravating/associated factors: food, activity, rest, certain movements; nausea, vomiting, diarrhea, fever, chills, etc.
  - Relieving factors: prescribed treatments and/or self-remedies, alternative or complementary therapies, their effect on the problem; food, rest, heat, ice, activity, position, etc.
  - Temporal factors: frequency; relation to other symptoms, problems, functions; symptom improvement or worsening over time
  - Severity of symptoms: quantify on a 0 (minimal) to 10 (severe) scale; effect on patient's lifestyle

MEDICAL HISTORY

- List and describe each of the following with dates of occurrence and any specific information available:
  - General health and strength over lifetime as patient perceives it; disabilities and functional limitations
  - Hospitalization and/or surgery: dates, hospital, diagnosis, complications
  - Injuries and disabilities
  - Major childhood illnesses
  - Adult illnesses and serious injuries
  - Immunizations: polio, diphtheria-pertussis-tetanus, tetanus toxoid, haemophilus influenza type b, hepatitis A and B, measles, mumps, rubella, varicella, Prevnar, influenza, anthrax, smallpox, cholera, typhus, typhoid, meningococcal, pneumococcal, bacille Calmette-Guérin, last purified protein derivative or other skin tests, unusual reaction to immunizations
  - Medications: past, current, recent medications (prescribed, nonprescription, complementary therapies, home remedies); dosages

- Allergies: drugs, foods, environmental
- Transfusions: reason, date, number of units transfused, reactions
- Emotional status: history of mood disorders, psychiatric attention or medications
- Recent laboratory tests (e.g., glucose, cholesterol, Pap smear, mammogram, prostate-specific antigen)

Family History

- Present information about age and health of family members in narrative or pedigree form, including at least three generations.
- Family members: Include parents, grandparents, aunts and uncles, siblings, spouse, children. For deceased family members, note age at time of death and cause, if known.
- Major health or genetic disorders: Include hypertension; cancer; cardiac, respiratory, kidney, or thyroid disorders; strokes; asthma or other allergic manifestations; blood dyscrasia; psychiatric difficulties; tuberculosis; diabetes mellitus; hepatitis; or other familial disorders. Note spontaneous abortions and stillbirths.

PERSONAL/SOCIAL HISTORY

- Include information according to concerns of patient and influence of health problem on patient's and family's life:
  - Cultural background and practices, birthplace, position in family
  - Marital status
  - Religious preference, religious or cultural proscriptions for medical care
  - Home conditions: economic condition, number in household, pets, presence of smoke detectors, presence and security of firearms
  - Occupation: work conditions and hours, physical or mental strain, protective devices used; exposure to chemicals, toxins, poisons, fumes, smoke, asbestos, or radioactive material at home or work
  - Environment: home, school, work; structural barriers if handicapped, community services utilized; travel; exposure to contagious diseases
  - Current health habits and/or risk factors: exercise; smoking; salt intake; weight control; dental hygiene diet, vitamins and other supplements; caffeine-containing beverages; alcohol or recreational drug use; response to CAGE, TACE, or RAFFT questions (see Appendix) related to alcohol use; participation in a drug or alcohol treatment program or support group
  - Sexual activity: protection method, contraception
  - General life satisfaction, hobbies, interests, sources of stress, adolescent's response to HEEADSSS questions (see Appendix)

REVIEW OF SYSTEMS

- Organize in general head-to-toe sequence, including an impression of each symptom.
- Record expected or negative findings as absence of symptoms or problems.
- When unexpected or positive findings are stated by patient, include details from further inquiry as you would in the present illness.
- Include the following categories of information (sequence may vary):
  - General constitutional symptoms
  - Diet
  - Skin, hair, nails
  - Head and neck
  - Eyes, ears, nose, mouth, throat
  - Endocrine
  - Breasts
  - Heart and blood vessels
  - Chest and lungs
  - Hematologic
  - Lymphatic, immunologic
  - Gastrointestinal
  - Genitourinary
  - Musculoskeletal
  - Neurologic
  - Psychiatric

OBJECTIVE DATA—PHYSICAL FINDINGS

Objective data are the findings resulting from direct observation—what you see, hear, and touch.

GENERAL STATEMENT

- Age, race, sex, general appearance
- Nutritional status, weight, height, frame size, body mass index
- Vital signs: temperature, pulse rate, respiratory rate, blood pressure (two extremities, two positions)

MENTAL STATUS

- Physical appearance and behavior
- Cognitive: memory, reasoning, attention span, response to questions
- Speech and language: voice quality, articulation, content, coherence, comprehension
- Emotional stability: anxiety, depression, disturbance in thought content

SKIN

- Color, integrity, temperature, hydration, tattoos, scars
- Presence of edema, excessive perspiration, unusual odor
- Presence and description of lesions (size, shape, location, inflammation, tenderness, induration, discharge), parasites
- Hair texture and distribution
- Nail configuration, color, texture, condition, presence of clubbing, nail plate adherence, firmness

HEAD

- Size and contour of head, scalp appearance and movement
- Facial features (characteristics, symmetry)
- Presence of edema or puffiness, tenderness
- Temporal arteries: characteristics

EYES

- Visual acuity, visual fields
- Appearance of orbits, conjunctivae, sclerae, eyelids, eyebrows
- Pupillary shape, consensual response to light and accommodation, extraocular movements, corneal light reflex, cover–uncover test
- Ophthalmoscopic findings of cornea, lens, retina, optic disc, macula, retinal vessel size, caliber, and arteriovenous crossings

EARS

- Configuration, position and alignment of auricles
- Otoscopic findings of canals (cerumen, lesions, discharge, foreign body) and tympanic membranes (integrity, color, landmarks, mobility, perforation)
- Hearing: air and bone conduction tests, whispered voice, conversation

NOSE

- Appearance of external nose, nasal patency, flaring
- Nasal mucosa and septum, color, alignment, discharge, crusting, polyp
- Appearance of turbinates
- Presence of sinus tenderness or swelling
- Discrimination of odors

MOUTH AND THROAT

- Number, occlusion and condition of teeth; presence of dental appliances
- Lips, tongue, buccal and oral mucosa, floor of mouth (color, moisture, surface characteristics, ulcerations, induration, symmetry)

- Oropharynx, tonsils, palate (color, symmetry, exudate)
- Symmetry and movement of tongue, soft palate and uvula; gag reflex
- Discrimination of taste

NECK

- Mobility, suppleness, strength
- Position of trachea
- Thyroid size, shape, tenderness, nodules
- Presence of masses, webbing, skinfolds

CHEST

- Size and shape of chest, anteroposterior versus transverse diameter, symmetry of movement with respiration
- Presence of retractions, use of accessory muscles, diaphragmatic excursion

LUNGS

- Respiratory rate, depth, regularity, quietness or ease of respiration
- Palpation findings: symmetry and quality of tactile fremitus, thoracic expansion
- Percussion findings: quality and symmetry of percussion notes, diaphragmatic excursion
- Auscultation findings: characteristics of breath sounds (pitch, duration, intensity, vesicular, bronchial, bronchovesicular), unexpected breath sounds
- Characteristics of cough
- Presence of friction rub, egophony, whispered pectoriloquy

BREASTS

- Size, contour, venous patterns
- Symmetry, texture, masses, scars, tenderness, thickening, nodules, discharge, retraction, or dimpling
- Characteristics of nipples and areolae

HEART

- Anatomic location of apical impulse
- Heart rate, rhythm, amplitude, contour
- Palpation findings: pulsations, thrills, heaves, or lifts
- Auscultation findings: characteristics of S_1 and S_2 (location, intensity, pitch, timing, splitting, systole, diastole)
- Presence of murmurs, clicks, snaps, S_3 or S_4 (timing, location, radiation intensity, pitch, quality)

BLOOD VESSELS

- Blood pressure: comparison between extremities with position change
- Jugular vein pulsations and distention, pressure measurement
- Presence of bruits over carotid, temporal, renal, and femoral arteries, abdominal aorta
- Pulses in distal extremities
- Temperature, color, hair distribution, skin texture, nail beds of lower extremities
- Presence of edema, swelling, vein distention, Homans sign, or tenderness of lower extremities

ABDOMEN

- Shape, contour, visible aorta pulsations, venous patterns, hernia
- Auscultation findings: bowel sounds in all quadrants, character
- Palpation findings: aorta, organs, feces, masses, location, size, contour, consistency, tenderness, muscle resistance
- Percussion findings: areas of different percussion notes, costovertebral angle tenderness
- Liver span

FEMALE GENITALIA

- Appearance of external genitalia and perineum, distribution of pubic hair, inflammation, excoriation, tenderness, scarring, discharge
- Internal examination findings: appearance of vaginal mucosa, cervix, discharge, odor, lesions
- Bimanual examination findings: size, position, tenderness of cervix, vaginal walls, uterus, adnexa, ovaries
- Rectovaginal examination findings
- Urinary incontinence with bearing down

MALE GENITALIA

- Appearance of external genitalia, circumcision status, location and size of urethral opening, discharge, lesions, distribution of pubic hair
- Palpation findings: penis, testes, epididymides, vasa deferentia, contour, consistency, tenderness
- Presence of hernia or scrotal swelling

ANUS AND RECTUM

- Sphincter control, presence of hemorrhoids, fissures, skin tags, polyps
- Rectal wall contour, tenderness, sphincter tone

- Prostate size, contour, consistency, mobility
- Color and consistency of stool

LYMPHATIC

- Presence of lymph nodes in head, neck, epitrochlear, axillary, or inguinal areas
- Size, shape, consistency, warmth, tenderness, mobility, discreteness of nodes

MUSCULOSKELETAL

- Posture: Alignment of extremities and spine, symmetry of body parts
- Symmetry of muscle mass, tone and muscle strength; grading of strength, fasciculations, spasms
- Range of motion, passive and active; presence of pain with movement
- Appearance of joints; presence of deformities, effusions, warmth, tenderness, or crepitus

NEUROLOGIC

- Cranial nerves: specific findings for each or specify those tested, if findings are recorded in head and neck sections
- Cerebellar and motor function: gait, balance, coordination with rapid alternating motions
- Sensory function, symmetry (touch, pain, vibration, temperature, monofilament)
- Superficial and deep tendon reflexes: symmetry, grade

ASSESSMENT

The assessment section is composed of your interpretations and conclusions, their rationale, the diagnostic possibilities, and present and anticipated problems—what you think.

For each new and existing problem on the problem list, make a differential diagnosis list with rationale based on subjective and objective data. Describe disease progression or complication.

PLAN

The plan describes the need to invoke diagnostic resources, therapeutic modalities, and other resources and the rationale for these decisions—what you intend to do.

- Diagnostic tests ordered or performed
- Therapeutic treatment plan
- Patient education
- Referrals initiated
- Future visit to evaluate plan

QUICK REFERENCE TO SPECIAL HISTORIES

CAGE Questionnaire: A Framework for Detecting Alcoholism

The CAGE questionnaire was developed in 1984 by Dr. John Ewing, and it
includes four interview questions designed to help diagnose alcoholism.
The acronym "CAGE" helps practitioners quickly recall the main concepts
of the four questions (**C**utting down, **A**nnoyance by criticism, **G**uilty feeling,
Eye-openers).

Probing questions may be asked as follow-up questions to the CAGE
questionnaire.

Many online resources list the complete questionnaire (e.g.,
http://addictionsandrecovery.org/addiction-self-test.htm). The exact
wording of the CAGE Questionnaire can be found in: Ewing JA: Screening
for Alcoholism using CAGE: cut down, annoyed, guilty, eye opener, *JAMA*
280(2): 1904-1905, 1984.

TACE Questionnaire: A Framework for Prenatal Detection of Risk Drinking

Mnemonic	Questions
T: Take	How many drinks does it take to make you feel high? (More than two drinks suggests a tolerance to alcohol that is a red flag.) How many when you first started drinking? When was that? Which do you prefer: beer, wine, or liquor?
A: Annoyed	Have people annoyed you by criticizing your drinking?
C: Cut down	Have you felt you ought to cut down on your drinking?
E: Eye-opener	Have you ever had an eye-opener drink first thing in the morning to steady your nerves or get rid of a hangover?

A positive answer to **T** alone or to two of **A, C,** or **E** may signal a problem with
a high degree of probability, and positive answers to all four, with great
certainty.

From Sokol et al, 1989.

The CRAFFT Questionnaire: A Framework for Detecting Recreational Substance Use Disorders in Adolescents

The CRAFFT questionnaire was developed in 2002 as a screening tool for alcohol and substance abuse in adolescents. The CRAFFT acronym helps practitioners remember the main concepts of the six questions: **C**ar, **R**elax, **A**lone, **F**orget, **F**riends, **T**rouble.

The exact wording of the CRAFFT questions can be found here: Knight JR et al., Validity of the CRAFFT Substance Abuse Screening Test Among Adolescent Clinic Patients. *Arch Pediatr Adolesc Med* 156:607-614, 2002 (available online at http://archpedi.jamanetwork.com/article.aspx?articleid=203511).

Domestic Violence: Three Questions as a Brief Screening Instrument

1. Have you been hit, kicked, punched, or otherwise hurt by someone within the past year?
2. Do you feel safe in your current relationship?
3. Is a partner from a previous relationship making you feel unsafe now?

A positive response to any one of the three questions constitutes a positive screen for partner violence.

The first question, which addresses physical violence, has been validated in studies as an accurate measure of 1-year prevalence rates.

The last two questions evaluate the perception of safety and estimate the short-term risk of further violence and the need for counseling, but reliability and validity evaluations have not yet been established.

From Feldhaus et al, 1997.

Brief Screening Tool for Domestic Violence: HITS

Verbal abuse is as intense a problem as physical violence. **HITS** stands for **H**urt, **I**nsult, **T**hreaten, or **S**cream. The wording of the question is, "In the last year, how often did your partner:

Hurt you physically?"
Insult or talk down to you?"
Threaten you with physical harm?"
Scream or curse at you?"

From Sherin et al, 1998.

BATHE Questionnaire: A Framework for Understanding the Patient in the Context of His or Her Total Life Situation

Mnemonic	Questions
B: Background	What is going on in your life?
	What is going on right now?
	Has anything changed recently?
A: Affect	How do you feel about that?
	What is your mood?
T: Trouble	What about the situation troubles you most?
	What worries or concerns you?
H: Handling	How are you handling that?
	How are you coping?
E: Empathy	That must be very difficult for you.
	I can understand that you would feel that way.

From Stuart and Lieberman, 1993; Lieberman, 1997.

HOPE Questionnaire: A Framework for Spiritual Assessment

Mnemonic	Questions
H: Hope—sources of hope, meaning, comfort, strength, peace, love, and connection	We have been discussing your support systems. I was wondering, what is there in your life that gives you internal support?
	What are your sources of hope, strength, comfort, and peace?
	What do you hold on to during difficult times?
	What sustains you and keeps you going?
	For some people, their religious or spiritual beliefs act as a source of comfort and strength in dealing with life's ups and downs; is this true for you?
	If the answer is yes, go on to **O** and **P** questions. If the answer is no, consider asking, "Was it ever?" If the answer is yes, ask, "What changed?"
O: Organized religion	Do you consider yourself part of an organized religion? How important is this to you?
	What aspects of your religion are helpful and not so helpful to you?
	Are you part of a religious or spiritual community? Does it help you? How?

HOPE Questionnaire: A Framework for Spiritual Assessment—cont'd

Mnemonic	Questions
P: Personal spirituality/practices	Do you have personal spiritual beliefs that are independent of organized religion? What are they? Do you believe in God? What kind of relationship do you have with God? What aspects of your spirituality or spiritual practices do you find most helpful to you personally? (Examples include prayer, meditation, reading scripture, attending religious services, listening to music, hiking, communing with nature.)
E: Effects on medical care and end-of-life issues	Has being sick (or your current situation) affected your ability to do the things that usually help you spiritually (or affected your relationship with God)? As a doctor, is there anything that I can do to help you access the resources that usually help you? Are you worried about any conflicts between your beliefs and your medical situation/care/decisions? Would it be helpful for you to speak to a clinical chaplain/community spiritual leader? Are there any specific practices or restrictions I should know about in providing your medical care (e.g., dietary restrictions, use of blood products)? If the patient is dying: How do your beliefs affect the kind of medical care you would like me to provide over the next few days/weeks/months?

From Anandarajah and Hight, 2001.

SPIRIT Questionnaire: A Framework for Spiritual Assessment

Mnemonic	Questions
S: Spiritual belief system	What is your formal religious affiliation?
	Name or describe your spiritual belief system.
P: Personal spirituality	Describe the beliefs and practices of your religion or spiritual system that you personally accept.
	Describe the beliefs or practices you do not accept.
	Do you accept or believe (specific tenet or practice)?
	What does your spirituality/religion mean to you?
	What is the importance of your spirituality/religion in daily life?
I: Integration with a spiritual community	Do you belong to any spiritual or religious group or community? What is your position or role?
	What importance does this group have to you? Is it a source of support? In what ways?
	Does or could this group provide help in dealing with health issues?
R: Ritualized practices and restrictions	Are there specific practices that you carry out as part of your religion/spirituality (e.g., prayer or meditation)?
	Are there certain lifestyle activities or practices that your religion/spirituality encourages or forbids? Do you comply?
	What significance do these practices and restrictions have to you?
	Are there specific elements of medical care that you forbid on the basis of religious/spiritual grounds?
I: Implications for medical care	What aspects of your religion/spirituality would you like me to keep in mind as I care for you?
	Would you like to discuss religious or spiritual implications of health care?
	What knowledge or understanding would strengthen our relationship as physician and patient?
	Are there any barriers to our relationship based on religious or spiritual issues?

SPIRIT Questionnaire: A Framework for Spiritual Assessment—cont'd

Mnemonic	Questions
T: Terminal events planning	As we plan for your care near the end of life, how does your faith affect your decisions? Are there particular aspects of care that you wish to forgo or have withheld because of your faith?

From Maugans, 1996.

ETHNIC Questionnaire: A Framework for Culturally Competent Clinical Practice

Mnemonic	Questions
E: Explanation	Why do you think you have these symptoms? What do friends, family, and others say? Do you know others with this problem? Have you seen it on TV, heard about it on the radio, or read about it in the newspaper?
T: Treatment	Do you take any treatments, medicines, or home remedies to treat the illness or to stay healthy? What kinds of treatment are you seeking from me?
H: Healers	Have you sought advice from friends, alternative folk healers, or other nondoctors?
N: Negotiate	Negotiate mutually acceptable options; incorporate patient's beliefs. Ask results patient hopes to achieve from intervention.
I: Intervention	Determine an intervention with your patient. May include incorporation of alternative treatments, spirituality, healers, or other cultural practices (e.g., foods to be eaten or avoided).
C: Collaborate	Collaborate with the patient, family, health team members, healers, and community resources.

Modified from Levin et al, 1997.

The HEEADSSS Psychosocial Interview for Adolescents (Essential Questions)

Mnemonic	Questions
H: Home	Who lives with you? Where do you live? Do you have your own room?
	What are relationships like at home?
	To whom are you closest at home?
	To whom can you talk at home?
	Is there anyone new at home? Has someone left recently?
	Have you moved recently?
	Have you ever had to live away from home? (Why?)
E: Education and employment	What are your favorite subjects at school?
	Your least favorite subjects?
	How are your grades? Any recent changes?
	Any dramatic changes in the past?
	Have you changed schools in the past few years?
	What are your future education/employment plans/goals?
	Are you working? Where? How much?
E: Eating	What do you like and not like about your body?
	Have there been any recent changes in your weight?
	Have you dieted in the last year? How? How often?
	Have you done anything else to try to manage your weight?
	How much exercise do you get in an average day? Week?
	What do you think would be a healthy diet?
	How does that compare to your current eating patterns?
A: Activities	What do you and your friends do for fun? (With whom, where, and when?)
	What do you and your family do for fun? (With whom, where, and when?)
	Do you participate in any sports or other activities?
	Do you regularly attend a church group, club, or other organized activity?
D: Drugs	Do you and your friends use tobacco? Alcohol? Other drugs?
	Does anyone in your family use tobacco? Alcohol? Other drugs?
	Do you use tobacco? Alcohol? Other drugs?
	Is there any history of alcohol or drug problems in your family? Does anyone at home use tobacco?

The HEEADSSS Psychosocial Interview for Adolescents (Essential Questions)—cont'd

Mnemonic	Questions
S: Sexuality	Have you ever been in a romantic relationship?
	Tell me about the people that you've dated. OR Tell me about your sex life.
	Have any of your relationships ever been sexual relationships?
	Are your sexual activities enjoyable?
	What does the term "safer sex" mean to you?
S: Suicide and depression	Do you feel sad or down more than usual?
	Do you feel yourself crying more than usual?
	Are you "bored" all the time?
	Are you having trouble getting to sleep?
	Have you thought a lot about hurting yourself or someone else?
S: Safety (savagery)	Have you ever been seriously injured? (How?) How about anyone else you know?
	Do you always wear a seatbelt in the car?
	Have you ever ridden with a driver who was drunk or high? When? How often?
	Do you use safety equipment for sports and/or other physical activities (e.g., helmets for biking or skateboarding)?
	Is there any violence at your school? In your neighborhood? Among your friends?
	Have you ever been physically or sexually abused? Have you ever been raped, on a date or at any other time? (if not asked previously)

From Goldenring and Rosen, 2004.

Adams JA: Evolution of a classification scale: medical evaluation of suspected child sexual abuse, *Child Maltreat* 6:31–36, 2001.

Agency for Healthcare Research and Quality: *Management of acute otitis media: summary, evidence report/technology assessment No. 15*, Rockville, Md, June 2000, Agency for Healthcare Research and Quality. www.ahrq.gov/clinic/epcsums/otitisum.htm (accessed 11/2005).

Ahuja V, et al: Head and neck manifestations of gastro-esophageal reflux disease, *Am Fam Physician* 50(3): 873–880, 885–886, 1999.

American Academy of Audiology: Newborn hearing screening. www.audiology.org/professional/tech/eihbrochure.php, 2002. (accessed 11/2005).

American Academy of Pediatrics: Committee on Bioethics: informed consent, parental permission, and assent in pediatric practice, *Pediatrics* 95(2):314–317, 1995.

American Academy of Pediatrics: Guidelines for the evaluation of sexual abuse of children: subject review (RE 9819), *Pediatrics* 103(1):186–191, 1999.

American Academy of Pediatrics and American Academy of Family Physicians: Clinical practice guideline: diagnosis and management of acute otitis media. www.aap.org/policy/otitis.htm, 2004. (accessed 11/2005).

American Academy of Pediatrics Committee on Quality Improvement, Subcommittee on Developmental Dysphasia of the Hip: Clinical practice guideline: early detection of developmental dysphasia of the hip, *Pediatrics* 105(4):896–905, 2000.

American Academy of Pediatrics Committee on Sports Medicine and Fitness: Medical conditions affecting sports participation, *Pediatrics* 107(5):1205–1209, 2001.

American Cancer Society: Cancer reference information: prevention and early detection. www.cancer.org (accessed 11/2013).

Anandarajah G, Hight E: Spirituality and medical practice: using the HOPE questions as a practical tool for spiritual assessment, *Am Fam Physician* 63(1):81–89, 2001.

Apantaku LM: Breast cancer diagnosis and screening, *Am Fam Physician* 62(3): 596–602, 2000.

Arvidson CR: The adolescent gynecologic exam,, *Pediatr Nurs* 25(1):71–74, 1999.

Athey J, Moody-Williams J: *Serving disaster survivors: achieving cultural competence in crisis counseling*, Washington, DC, 2000, Emergency Services and Disaster Relief Branch, Center for Mental Health Services, Substance Abuse and Mental Health Services Administration.

Attia MW, et al: Performance of a predictive model for streptococcal pharyngitis in children, *Arch Pediatr Adolesc Med* 155:687–691, 2001.

Bacal DA, Wilson MC: Strabismus: getting it straight, *Contemp Pediatr* 17:49, 2000.

Baran R, et al: *Color atlas of the hair, scalp and nails*, St Louis, 1991, Mosby.

Barkauskas VH, et al: *Health and physical assessment*, ed 3, St Louis, 2002, Mosby.

Bastiaens L, et al: The RAFFT as a screening tool for adolescent substance use disorders,, *Am J Addict* 9(1):10–16, 2000.

Bluestone CD, Klein JO: *Otitis media in infants and children*, ed 3, Philadelphia, 2001, Saunders.

Boustani M, et al: Screening for dementia in primary care: a summary of the evidence for the U.S. Preventive Services Task Force, *Ann Intern Med* 138:927–937, 2003.

Brooke P, Bullock R: Validation of a 6-item cognitive impairment test with a view to primary care, *Int J Geriatr Psychiatry* 14(1):936–940, 1999.

Brown JE, Carlson M: Nutrition and multi-fetal pregnancy, *J Am Diet Assoc* 100(3):343–348, 2000.

Burrow GN: Thyroid diseases. In Burrow GN, Duffy TP, editors: *Medical complications during pregnancy*, ed 6, Philadelphia, 2004, Saunders.

Castiglia PT: Depression in children, *J Pediatr Health Care* 14(2):73–75, 2000.

Caulin-Glaser T, Setaro J: Pregnancy and cardiovascular disease. In Burrow GN, Duffy TP, editors: *Medical complications during pregnancy*, ed 6, Philadelphia, 1999, Saunders.

Centers for Disease Control and Prevention: 2007 Guideline for Isolation Precautions: Preventing Transmission of Infectious Agents in Healthcare Settings. http://www.cdc.gov/ncidod/dhqp/pdf/isolation2007.pdf (accessed 11/2013).

Centers for Disease Control and Prevention: Healthcare Infection Control Practices Advisory Committee (HICPAC). http://www.cdc.gov/hicpac/2007IP/2007ip_part3.html (accessed 11/2013).

Centers for Disease Control and Prevention: Viral hepatitis. www.cdc.gov/ncidod/diseases/hepatitis/index.htm (accessed 11/2005).

Chelebowski RT, et al: Influence of estrogen plus progestin on breast cancer and mammography in healthy postmenopausal women: the Woman's Health Initiative randomized trial, *JAMA* 289:3243–3253, 2003.

Chopard G, Pitard A, Ferreira S, Vanholsbeeck G, Rumbach L, Galmiche J: Combining the Memory Impairment Screen and the Isaacs Set Test: a practical tool for screening dementias, *J Am Geriatr Soc* 55(9):1426–1430, 2007.

Chumlea W, et al: Age at menarche and racial comparisons in U.S. girls, *Pediatrics* 111:110–113, 2003; www.pediatrics.org/cgi/content/full/111/1/110 (accessed 11/2005).

D'Arcy CA, McGee S: Does this patient have carpal tunnel syndrome? *JAMA* 283(23):3110–3117, 2000.

Dains J, et al: *Advanced health assessment & clinical diagnosis in primary care*, ed 4, Philadelphia, 2011, Mosby.

Deering CG: To speak or not to speak: self-closure with patients, *Am J Nurs* 99:34–38, 1999.

Delves PJ, Roitt IM: The immune system, *N Engl J Med* 343:108–116, 2000.

Doerflinger DMC: The Mini-Cog,, *Am J Nurs* 107(12):62–71, 2007.

Dowd R, Cavalieri RJ: Help your patient live with osteoporosis, *Am J Nurs* 99(4):55–60, 1999.

Edge V, Miller M: *Women's health care*, St Louis, 1994, Mosby.

Ewing JA: Screening for alcoholism using CAGE: cut down, annoyed, guilty, eye opener, *JAMA* 280(2):1904–1905, 1998.

Executive Summary of the Third Report of the National Cholesterol Education Program Expert Panel on Detection, Evaluation, and Treatment of High Blood Cholesterol in Adults (Adult Treatment Panel III), *JAMA* 285(19):2486–2497, 2001.

Farrar WE, et al: *Infectious diseases*, ed 2, London, 1992, Gower.

Fedarko NS: The biology of aging and frailty, *Clin Geriatr Med* 27(1):27–37, 2011.

Feldhaus K, et al: Accuracy of 3 brief screening questions for detecting partner violence in the emergency department, *JAMA* 277(17):1357–1361, 1997.

Ferrie B: Complementary modalities in the new millennium, *Adv Nurs May* 3:28–29, 1999.

Ferro RT, et al: A nonoperative approach to shoulder impingement syndrome, *Adv Stud Med* 3(9):518–528, 2003.

Folstein M, et al: The meaning of cognitive impairment in the elderly, *J Am Geriatr Soc* 33(4):228, 1985.

Folstein MF, et al: "Mini-Mental State": a practical method for grading the cognitive state of patients for the clinician, *J Psychiatr Res* 12:189, 1975.

Franklin SS, et al: Is pulse pressure useful in prediction risk for coronary heart disease? *Circulation* 100:354, 1999.

Frisancho AR: New norms of upper limb fat and muscle areas for assessment of nutritional status, *Am J Clin Nutr* 34:2540, 1981.

Frisancho AR: New standards of weight and body composition by frame size and height for assessment of nutritional status of adults and the elderly, *Am J Clin Nutr* 40:808, 1984.

Frisch RE: Growth Diagrams 1965 Netherlands: Second National Survey on 0-24-Year-Olds, by J. C. Van Wieringen et al, *Pediatrics* 49:484–485, 1972.

Gardosi J, Francis A: Controlled trial of fundal height measurement plotted on customized antenatal growth charts, *Br J Obstet Gynecol* 104(4):309–317, 1999.

Goldenring JM, Rosen DS: Getting into adolescent heads: an essential update, *Contemp Pediatr* 21(1):64–90, 2004.

Goldman MP, Fitzpatrick RE: *Cutaneous laser surgery: the art and science of selective photothermolysis*, ed 2, St Louis, 1999, Mosby.

Grundy S, et al: Implications of recent clinical trials for the National Cholesterol Education Program Adult Treatment Panel III Guidelines, *Circulation* 110:227–239, 2004; http://circ.ahajournals.org/ (accessed 12/2005).

Habif TP: *Clinical dermatology*, ed 5, St Louis, 2010, Mosby.

Haller CA, Benowitz NL: Adverse cardiovascular and central nervous system events associated with dietary supplements containing ephedra alkaloids, *N Engl J Med* 343:1833–1842, 2000.

Hardie GE, et al: Ethnic descriptors used by African-American and white asthma patients during induced bronchoconstriction, *Chest* 117:935–943, 2000.

Harvey AM, et al: *The principles and practice of medicine*, ed 22, Norwalk, CT, 1988, Appleton & Lange.

Hennigan L, et al: Methods for managing pelvic examination anxiety: individual differences and relaxation techniques, *J Pediatr Health Care* 14(1):9–12, 2000.

Hoberman A, Paradise JL: Acute otitis media: diagnosis and management in the year 2000, *Pediatr Ann* 29(10):609–620, 2000.

Hockenberry MJ, Wilson D: *Wong's essentials of pediatric nursing*, ed 9, St Louis, 2013, Mosby.

Hockenberry MJ, Wilson D: *Wong's nursing care of infants and children*, ed 9, St Louis, 2011, Mosby.

Hockenberry M, Wilson D: *Wong's nursing care of infants and children*, ed 8, St Louis, 2007, Mosby.

Hornor G: Sexual behavior in children: normal or not? *J Pediatr Health Care* 18(2):57–64, 2004 Mar-Apr.

Jacobson A: Research for practice: saving limbs with Semmes-Weinstein monofilament, *Am J Nurs* 99(2):76, 1999.

Jacobson RD: Approach to the child with weakness and clumsiness, *Pediatr Clin North Am* 45(1):145–168, 1998.

James WD, Berger TG, Elson DM: *Andrew's diseases of the skin: clinical dermatology*, ed 10, London, WB Saunders, 2000.

Jerant AF, et al: Early detection and treatment of skin cancer, *Am Fam Physician* 62(2):357–368, 375-376, 381–382, 2000.

Johnson TS, et al: Reliability of three length measurement techniques in term infants, *Pediatr Nurs* 25(1):13–17, 1999.

Judge R, et al: *Clinical diagnosis*, ed 5, Boston, 1988, Little, Brown.

Kass-Wolff J, Wilson E: Pediatric gynecology: assessment strategies and common problems, *Semin Reprod Med* 21(4):329–338, 2003.

Kellogg N: American Academy of Pediatrics Committee on Child Abuse and Neglect, American Academy of Pediatrics: The evaluation of sexual abuse in children, *Pediatrics* 116(2):506–512, 2005.

Kerker BD, et al: Identification of violence in the home, *Arch Pediatr Adolesc Med* 154:457–462, 2000.

Kernan WN, et al: Phenylpropanolamine and risk of hemorrhagic stroke, *N Engl J Med* 343:1826–1832, 2000.

Khandker RK, et al: A decision model and cost-effectiveness analysis of colorectal cancer screening and surveillance guidelines for average-risk adults, *Int J Technol Assess Health Care* 16(3):799–810, 2000.

Knight JR, et al: A new brief screen for adolescent substance abuse, *Arch Pediatr Adolesc Med* 153:591–596, 1999.

Knight JR, et al: Reliabilities of short substance-abuse screening tests among adolescent medical patients, *Pediatrics* 105:948–953, 2000.

Koop CE: *The Surgeon General's letter on child sexual abuse*, Rockville, Md, 1988, U.S. Department of Health and Human Services.

Koopman WJ, Moreland LW: *Arthritis and allied conditions: a textbook of rheumatology*, ed 15, Philadelphia, 2004, Lippincott Williams & Wilkins.

Kuczmarski MF, et al: Descriptive anthropometric reference data for older Americans, *J Am Diet Assoc* 100:59–66, 2000.

Lanham DM, et al: Accuracy of tympanic temperature readings in children under 6 years of age, *Pediatr Nurs* 25(1):39–42, 1999.

Lapinsky S: Cardiopulmonary changes in pregnancy: what you need to know, *Women's Health in Primary Care* 2:353, 1999.

Lehne R: *Pharmacology for nursing care*, ed 8, St Louis, 2013, Saunders.

Lemmi FO, Lemmi CAE: *Physical assessment findings CD-ROM*, Philadelphia, 2000, Saunders.

Levin SJ, et al: ETHNIC: A framework for culturally competent clinical practice,, *Patient Care* 9(special issue):188, 2000.

Lieberman JA: III: BATHE: an approach to the interview process in the primary care setting, *J Clin Psychiatry* 58(Suppl 3):3–6, 1997.

Lipman TH, et al: Assessment of growth by primary health care providers, *J Pediatr Health Care* 14(4):166–171, 2000.

Lowdermilk DL, Perry SE: *Maternity and women's health care*, ed 8, St Louis, 2004, Mosby.

Lowdermilk DL, Perry SE: *Maternity and women's health care*, ed 10, St Louis, 2012, Mosby.

Maron BJ, et al: Recommendations and considerations related to preparticipation screening for cardiovascular abnormalities in competitive athletes: 2007 update: a scientific statement from the American Heart Association Council on Nutrition, Physical Activity, and Metabolism: endorsed by the American College of Cardiology Foundation, *Circulation* 115(12):1643–1655, 2007.

Maslow K, Mezey M: Recognition of dementia in hospitalized older adults, *Am J Nurs* 108(1):40–49, 2008.

Mattson JE: The language of pain, *Reflections on Nursing Leadership* Fourth quarter:11–14, 2000.

Maynard CK: Differentiate depression from dementia, *Nurse Pract* 28(3):18–27, 2003.

Maugans TA: The SPIRITual history, *Arch Fam Med* 5(1):11–16, 1996.

McCaffery M, Pasero C: Teaching patients to use a numerical pain-rating scale, *Am J Nurs* 99:22, 1999.

McCarty DJ: *Arthritis and allied conditions: a textbook of rheumatology*, ed 12, Philadelphia, 1993, Lea & Febiger.

McClain N, et al: Evaluation of sexual abuse in the pediatric patient, *J Pediatr Health Care* 14(3):93–102, 2000.

McNeese M: Evaluation of sexual abuse in the pediatric patient, *J Pediatr Health Care* 14(3):93–102, 2000.

Miyasaki-Ching CM: *Chasteen's essentials of clinical dental assisting*, ed 5, St Louis, 1997, Mosby.

Moody CW: Male child sexual abuse, *J Pediatr Health Care* 13:112–119, 1999.

Morrow M: The evaluation of common breast problems, *Am Fam Physician* 61(8):2371–2378, 2385, 2000.

Moyer LA, et al: Hepatitis C: Part II. Prevention counseling and medical evaluation, *Am Fam Physician* 59(2):349–354, 357, 1999.

National Cholesterol Education Program Expert Panel on Detection: Evaluation, and Treatment of High Blood Cholesterol in Adults: Executive summary of the third report of the National Cholesterol Education Program (NCEP) Expert Panel on Detection, Evaluation, and Treatment of High Blood Cholesterol (Adult Treatment Panel III), *JAMA* 285(19):2486–2497, 2001.

National Institutes of Health: Report No. 48–4080, Bethesda, Md, 1997, National Institutes of Health.

Naway H, et al: Concordance of clinical findings and clinical judgment in diagnosis of streptococcal pharyngitis, *Acad Emerg Med* 7(10):1104–1109, 2000.

Nuss R, Manco-Johnson MJ: Venous thrombosis: issues for the pediatrician, *Contemp Pediatr* 17:75, 2000.

Patton KT, Thibodeau GA: *Anatomy & physiology*, ed 8, St Louis, 2013, Mosby.

Pletcher SD: Goldberg: The diagnosis and treatment of sinusitis, *Adv Stud Med* 3(9):495–506, 2003.

Ramsburg KL: Rheumatoid arthritis, *AJN Am J Neuroradiol* 100(11): 40–43, 2000.

Rockwood K, Mitnitski A: Frailty defined by deficit accumulation and geriatric medicine defined by frailty, *Clin Geriatr Med* 27(1):17–26, 2011.

Rosenthal TC, Puck SM: Screening for genetic risk of breast cancer, *Am Fam Physician* 59(1):99–104, 106, 1999.

Samiy AH, et al: *Textbook of diagnostic medicine*, Philadelphia, 1987, Lea & Febiger.

Schulman KA, et al: The effects of race and sex on physicians' recommendations for cardiac catheterization,, *N Engl J Med* 340:618–626, 1999.

Scott M, Gelhot AR: Gastroesophageal reflux disease: diagnosis and management, *Am Fam Physician* 59(5):1161–1169, 1199, 1999.

Sheikh JL, Yesavage JA: Geriatric depression scale: recent evidence and development of a shorter version, *Clin Gerontol* 5:165–172, 1986.

Shinitzky HE, Kub J: The art of motivating behavior change: the use of motivational interviewing to promote health, *Pub Health Nurs* 18:178–185, 2001.

Sloan RP, et al: Should physicians prescribe religious activities? *N Engl J Med* 342:1913–1916, 2000.

Smith RD, McNamara JJ: The neurological examination of children with school problems, *J Sch Health* 54(7):231–234, 1984.

Sokol RJ, et al: TACE questions: practical prenatal detection of risk-drinking, *Am J Obstet Gynecol* 260(4):863–868, 1989.

Starr NB, et al: Malocclusion: how important is that bite? *J Pediatr Health Care* 13:245–247, 1999.

Stuart MR, Lieberman III JA: *The fifteen-minute hour: applied psychotherapy for the primary care physician*, ed 2, New York, 1993, Praeger.

Teoh TG, Fisk NM: Hydramnios, oligohydramnios. In James DK, et al: *High-risk pregnancy: management options*, ed 2, Philadelphia, 1999, Saunders.

Thomas AE, et al: A nomogram method for assessing body weight,, *Am J Clin Nutr* 29(3):302–304, 1976.

Thompson JM, et al: *Mosby's clinical nursing*, ed 4, St Louis, 1997, Mosby.

Thompson JM, et al: *Mosby's clinical nursing*, ed 5, St Louis, 2002, Mosby.

U.S. Department of Agriculture: MyPyramid. www.mypyramid.gov (accessed Nov. 30, 2005).

U.S. Preventive Services Task Force: *Guide to clinical preventive services*, 2012, U.S. Government Printing Office. http://www.ahrq.gov/professionals/clinicians-providers/guidelines-recommendations/guide/index.html (accessed 11/2013, 2005).

U.S. Preventive Services Task Force: *Recommendations*, http://www.uspreventiveservices taskforce.org/recommendations.htm (accessed 11/2013).

Van Wieringen JC, Wafelbakker F, Verbrugge HP, DeHaas JH. Groningen: Noordhoff Uitgevers BV: *Growth diagrams 1965 Netherlands: second national survey on 0-24-year-olds*, The Netherlands.

Varcarolis EM: *Psychiatric nursing clinical guide: assessment tools and diagnosis*, Philadelphia, 1999, Saunders.

Videlefsky A, et al: Routine vaginal cuff smear testing in post-hysterectomy patients with benign uterine conditions: when is it indicated? *J Am Board Fam Pract* 13(4):233–238, 2000.

Warner PH, et al: Shedding light on the sexual history, *AJN Am J Neuroradiol* 99:34–40, 1999.

Werk LN, et al: Medicine for the millennium: demystifying EBM, *Contemp Pediatr* 16:87–107, 1999.

Weston WL, Lane AT: *Color textbook of pediatric dermatology*, St Louis, 1991, Mosby.

Weston WL, Lane AT, Mortelli JG: *Color textbook of pediatric dermatology*, ed 2, St Louis, 1996, Mosby.

Weston WL, et al: *Color textbook of pediatric dermatology*, ed 4, St Louis, 2007, Mosby.

White GM: *Color atlas of regional dermatology*, St Louis, 1994, Mosby.

Whooley MA, Simon GE: Managing depression in medical outpatients, *N Engl J Med* 343:1942–1950, 2000.

Wilson MEH: Keeping quiet, *Arch Pediatr Adolesc Med* 152:1054–1055, 1999.

Wilson SF, Giddens JF: *Health assessment for nursing practice*, ed 5, St Louis, 2013, Mosby.

Wright RJ: Identification of violence in the community pediatric setting, *Arch Pediatr Adolesc Med* 154:431–433, 2000.

Zitelli BJ, McIntire SC, Nowalk AJ: *Zitelli and Davis': Atlas of pediatric physical diagnosis*, ed 6, St Louis, 2013, Mosby.

Page numbers followed by *f* indicate figures; *t*, tables; *b*, boxes.

313

INDEX